PRIVATISATION AND THE NATIONAL HEALTH SERVICE

Privatisation and the National Health Service

The Scope for Collaboration

JEFF CHANDRA
and
ANDREW KAKABADSE
Cranfield School of Management
Cranfield Institute of Technology

Avebury

Aldershot · Brookfield USA · Hong Kong · Singapore · Sydney

Published by
Avebury
Gower Publishing Company Limited
Gower House
Croft Road
Aldershot
Hants GU11 3HR
England

Gower Publishing Company
Old Post Road
Brookfield
Vermont 05036
USA

Reprinted 1987

British Library Cataloguing in Publication Data
Chandra, Jeff
Privatisation and the National Health Service :
the scope for collaboration.
1. Great Britain----National Health Service
2. Medical care----Great Britain 3. Medical care,
Cost of----Great Britain
I. Title II. Kakabadse, Andrew
362.1'0941 RA395.G6

ISBN 0 566 00813 0

Printed in Great Britain by
Antony Rowe Limited, Chippenham, Wiltshire.

Contents

Acknowledgements		vii
	CHAPTER	
1	Scope of the Study	1
2	What is Privatisation?	3
3	Intermesh between the NHS and the Private Sector	9
4	Origins, Size and Growth of the Health Care Industry	21
5	Arguments for and against Private Medicine	35
6	Case Studies in Privatisation	47
7	Towards Collaboration at the Local Level	65
8	Summary of Possible Actions for the NHS	73
References		76
	APPENDICES	
1	Changes Planned Towards Privatisation	78
2	Amenity and Private Beds in England	79
3	Hospital and Community Service: Contracting Out (England 1980/81)	80
4	BUPA, PPP, WPA - Key Statistics	81
5	Main Points from 1981 Reports and Accounts of Health Insurance Companies	82
6	1982 NALGO Annual Conference Resolution on Private Medicine	83
7	Advertisement by Independent Hospital Unit	84

Appendices contd

8 Letter from Minister of Health to Chairmen of Health Authorities - 20 August 1981 85

9 Extract from Paper on Contracting Out Cleaning Services in District X. 87

Acknowledgements

A considerable volume of material in this study relates to events in a particular NHS Health District. The Authors would like to extend their gratitude to the District Administrator for making information freely available at all times.

Many thanks also to Mairi Bryce for her high standard of work on the word processor, and patience and understanding in having to alter draft after draft to suit the authors' requirements.

1 Scope of the study

Introduction

In a recent article in the Health and Social Services Journal, Raymond Kirk (1982), a consultant surgeon, said:

> 'Discussion of private practice and socialised medicine is not a matter of marshalling facts and figures alone. It is among the many contentious issues of moral and social philosophy. On the one hand there are those who believe that to create an egalitarian world all forms of privilege should be barred and two important targets are private medicine and private education. In opposition to that view is the deeply held belief in individual freedom to pursue one's own activities provided that they do no harm to the rest of population.'

The article is one of many which have appeared in recent years, and particularly since the issue of privatisation became a major plank in the economic and social policies pursued by the Conservative Governments elected in 1979 and 1983. Throughout the process of 'insidious encroachment' by the private medical industry (as some would call it) or 'bold initiatives' (as others see it) the National Health Service (NHS) has been, at best, ambiguous about its posture towards this growing phenomenon.

Threats for the NHS

The fundamental assumption underlying this study is that the present ambiguous and apparently passive stance of the NHS in relation to the private medical sector is no longer tenable. The primary reason for this is that there is a very real danger that a 'head-in-the-sand' strategy could lead to the very mode which the NHS fears most - the provider of second class services to second class citizens. It will be evident from this assumption that the perspective taken for the study relates to the possible strategies the NHS might adopt in the face of a changing environment.

Scope of the Debate

However, as Raymond Kirk has suggested, the canvas for the debate about privatisation in health care is vast. At one extreme the debate must encompass the philosophy and value systems which govern the organisation of society now and in the future. At the other extreme the debate could relate to financial comparisons between each element of public and privately provided medical services. Somewhere in the middle would come the managerial perspectives which relate to competitive strategy for organisations, economic theories of market behaviour,the management of change in organisations, and management of inter-organisational relations to name but a few.

Scope of the Study

A study such as this would not be complete unless it recognised all the above dimensions. However, the corollary is that there is no single theoretical model which could be adopted against which to analyse the NHS as part of a changing medical care industry or one which would yield strategies capable of implementation on a broad front in the future. The approach which has therefore been adopted is a pragmatic one, designed to be of practical value to those in the NHS who know little about the health care industry as a whole (the overwhelming majority) and the few who carry the responsibility for guiding the fortunes of the NHS.

Chapter 2: Analysis of the concept of 'privatisation' and in particular how the concept relates to the NHS.

Chapter 3: Discussion of the numerous points of contact which already exist between the State and private sectors of medicine.

Chapter 4: Examination of the present size of the public and private medical care sectors and growth prospects.

Chapter 5: Discussion of the arguments for and against privatisation in medical care.

Chapter 6: Case studies relating to the response of one NHS District to the pressure to 'privatise'.

Chapter 7: Possible ways in which the NHS at local level might regain the initiative in the privatisation issue.

Chapter 8: Summary of ways in which the NHS might deal with privatisation, keeping the pros and cons in mind.

2 What is privatisation?

Post War Consensus

The Public Sector in Britain grew in leaps and bounds after the second world war. During the post war reconstruction the Labour Government (1945-1951) embarked on a large scale programme of nationalisation of the country's basic industries - coal, railways, steel and airlines - some of which were termed the 'commanding heights of the economy'. The National Health Service came into being in 1948 as part of the thinking that these vital industries and sevices were of too great a strategic or social importance to be left to the vagaries of the market place. No doubt the traumatic experience of the 1930s and the war itself contributed towards the post war consensus about the role of the public sector.

Whilst governments of both political complexions during the 1950s and 1960s maintained state control over these industries and services, it was the Labour government of 1974-1979 which gave a further impetus to nationalisation, for example with the establishment of the National Enterprise Board (NEB), which brought many firms under public ownership and control.

Changing Times

The Conservative Government elected in 1979 claimed a mandate for rolling back the frontiers of public ownership and this date perhaps marks the major break from the consensus politics of previous years. Whilst proclaiming a commitment to the welfare state the government has set its major objections as beating inflation through monetary policy, requiring, in particular, tight control of the Public Sector Borrowing Requirement (PSBR). The policy has obvious implications for publicly financed industries and services. But in addition, the Conservatives, as a party of free enterprise, have a keen ideological commitment to a reduction of the State's role in the economy, together with creating a climate in which the private sector can flourish. Sir Geoffrey Howe, former Chancellor of the Exchequer, summarised the government's attitude to public sector enterprises as follows:

> 'A private firm must adapt its production - in quality, specification, cost and volume - to what the

consumer will buy, or go out of business. The consumer is sovereign in the private sector. In the public sector he is dethroned by subsidy or monopoly'.

So what steps does the Government intend in order to restore the supremacy of the consumer - to 'privatise' as the process has become known? The three basic mechanisms are set out below and Appendix I identifies the elements of 'privatisation' as they apply to a number of companies and industries.

Selling off Public Assets

The government can sell to the private sector any assets it holds. These may include shares or real assets such as land and property. The government have effected a number of such disposals and declared plans for other firms and industries. For example:

British Petroleum. In January 1980 the government sold 5 per cent of its holdings for £270 million, reducing its share of the total capital to 44.6 per cent.

National Enterprise Board. The NEB was instructed to sell off all its holdings as soon as possible. The most important sales were: ICL for £37 million; Ferranti for £54 million and Fairey's for £22 million.

British Aerospace. In February 1981 the government sold shares and it now has only 48 per cent of the holding.

Cable and Wireless. In October 1981, nearly 50 per cent of the shares were sold for £22 million.

National Freight Corporation. In January 1982, it was agreed to sell off £53.5 million of NFC shares.

British Rail. Some of the BR hotels have already been sold off and BR Hoverspeed has merged with the privately owned Hoverlloyd.

Amersham International. The government sold a large share of the capital of the radio-chemical firm in February 1982 amidst a public outcry. The shares sold for a total of £71 million, and immediately after the sale were priced by the stock market at £97 million.

Forestry Commission. The government intends to sell large areas of Forestry Commission land. It has already sold off The Stang, a 1,500 acre woodland area in County Durham to an unknown buyer at an unknown price. It is speculated that the probable purchaser is an institution such as a pension fund which sees the woodland giving a dependable long term return.

British National Oil Corporation. Legislation, enabling the oil production and exploration work of the British National Oil Corporation (BNOC) to be sold on the market, is to be passed through Parliament. The government hopes that it will be able to raise £600-£700 million from the sale of these assets over the next two years.

British Gas. Shares are to be sold off, notably the 50 per cent stake in the Wytch Oil Farm, despite vigorous opposition from British Gas itself. In March 1983 a fierce controversy raged about the price which the shares should fetch.

British Telecom. The government is considering the sale of shares.

British Transport Docks Board. The government has plans to sell off 49 per cent of the shares as soon as possible.

British Airways. The government is committed to selling shares, but the original target date of early 1983 has been postponed so that the airline can be 'nursed' back to financial health to make it attractive to the market, a policy which is succeeding.

Creating New Markets for the Private Sector

In those industries where the government does not intend to sell off public assets, it may seek to change the conditions under which they operate. Essentially, this involves the government forcing public enterprise to behave more in line with firms in the private sector, a particular target being the State monopolies.

To further buttress its policy of privatisation the government in 1980 introduced the Competition Act which gives it the power - through the Monopolies and Mergers Commission - to investigate nationalised industry monopolies. The Commission has already produced seven reports suggesting improvements in the running of each industry. Some of the major outcomes have been as follows:

Post Office/British Telecom. The 1981 Telecommunications Act ended the monopoly position of the Post Office and British Telecom in respect of some of their services. The Act also gives the Secretary of State the power to make further relaxations. A number of companies, including the consortium involving Cable and Wireless and Barclay's Bank (the 'Mercury Project'), are bidding strongly in the market for the highly profitable 'privatised' business.

Electricity. The government plans to introduce legislation abolishing the Central Electricity Generating Board's monopoly of the generation of electricity. Competition would be allowed by ending the ban on the private production and sale of electricity as a main business.

British Gas. British Gas is to lose its monoposonistic position as a buyer of indigenous gas. This will be opened up to private enterprise.

National Bus. Private companies were encouraged under the 1980 Transport Act to set up in competition to the National Bus Company.

Encouragement to 'Opt Out'

A number of the measures taken by the government have the strategic objective of encouraging the development of the private sector of services presently provided by public bodies. The strategy can take two complementary forms. Firstly, the government can take active steps to encourage individuals to 'opt out' of publicly provided services and, secondly, it can withhold the finance necessary for public services to meet the demands being placed on them. Examples of the first include the tax relief provided on private health insurance premiums to those individuals earning less than £8,500 per annum, and increased charges for public services e.g. bus fares, school meals and NHS prescriptions. An example of the second is the withholding of resources necessary to meet increased demands for services. For example, the NHS needs growth of some 1 per cent per annum just to meet the extra demands due to demographic changes (such as the rising number of elderly people), let alone to improve services. Both these sorts of measures contribute to dissatisfaction with public sector services and the creation of demand which the private sector is encouraged to meet.

Privatisation in Local Government

The process of privatisation in local government and the National Health Service is intended to take a number of forms.

External Audit. Each Local Authority has its own internal audit to ensure appropriate use of public and ratepayers' funds. The government does not accept that the internal auditing function has been strong enough and has established the Audit Commission which has the duty to investigate whether the local authority is providing value for money.

Contracting Out. Some of the Conservative controlled Local Authorities wish to encourage the 'contracting out' of services previously provided in-house. These services include catering, laundry, cleaning, transport, printing, security, purchasing of supplies, building maintenance and repairs, management services etc. In many ways the growth in local government manpower is one of the easiest political targets, and one which unites ratepayers and taxpayers alike. Anecdotes of Town Hall waste and extravagance are legion. The following indicates the level of local government manpower nationally in some of the services mooted for contracting out:

170,000	in Direct Labour Organisations (concerned with building and housing maintenance)
46,000	in refuse collection and cleansing
36,000	in cleaning local government premises
134,000	school cleaners.

In 1980 the Local Government Planning and Land Act became law. The main aim of the Act was to force Direct Labour Organisations (DLOs) to compete with private firms. The Act requires open tendering for all work valued above an amount laid down by the Secretary of State for the Environment (currently £10,000 per job), and as of 1 October 1982, for 30 per cent of works of maintenance below that threshold. The Act also requires all DLOs to keep separate accounts for different areas of work (highways, new work and maintenance) and to publish such accounts in the traditional business accounting formats of Balance sheets and Profit and Loss Accounts. The main objectives are seen by some cynics as not being particularly beneficial to local government Councillors, management, employees or tenants, but as vital business information for private companies contemplating competitive tendering.

Privatisation in the National Health Service

It is important to recognise that the government's proposals on privatisation in the NHS encompass all the main elements of the strategy identified in earlier paragraphs, namely:

<u>Selling off assets</u>: The NHS is required to keep in mind the possibility that a private hospital developer might wish to purchase redundant NHS property or buildings.

<u>Creating New Markets</u>: As in local government, health authorities have an internal audit function and their accounts are also audited by DHSS. The government, however, remains convinced that the accounts should be audited 'externally' and, for example, has commissioned Coopers and Lybrand to undertake an audit of Ealing Health Authority accounts. Again as in local government, the government has made clear its intention to see a major shift towards the 'contracting out' of clinical and 'hotel' services currently provided within the NHS.

Encouragement to 'Opt Out': Reference has already been made to the incentive of tax relief now being offered to those earning less than £8,500 p.a. to take out private health insurance. In addition, there is a considerable body of opinion which believes that the NHS is being deliberately starved of the resources it needs to meet the demands being placed upon it, thus generating a level of dissatisfaction with the services provided.

Whilst all three elements of the privatisation strategy are relevant for the NHS, the above broad framework does not reflect the extremely close inter-relationships between the public and private sectors of medicine. It is important to appreciate the points of contact in order to ascertain whether recent government initiatives are merely the extension of existing principles and practices or a radical departure from the status quo in 1979. It is this issue which is addressed in the next Chapter.

3 Intermesh between the NHS and the private sector

The issue about the respective roles of the public and private sectors of health care has risen rapidly on the political agenda over the last few years. As the debate has gained momentum following the election of a Conservative Government in 1979, a number of the protagonists have adopted and publicised their respective positions. The battle lines are now clearly drawn and are analysed in some detail in Chapter 5.

The current high profile of this debate often gives the misleading impression that the health care industry is a virtually 100 per cent State monopoly. The impression is misleading because the reality is that in virtually every aspect of the industry the non-state sector has played a role for decades. The role has varied from a notional presence, as in the case of private general practitioners, to the case where virtually all the pharmaceutical product requirements of the industry are met by the private sector. This Section examines the subtle and the obvious inter-relationships between the State and independent sectors in the health care industry, demonstrates the long standing nature of the relationships and identifies the crucial dependence of one sector on the other.

Supply of Goods and Materials

The NHS relies on the private sector almost totally for supplies of goods and materials - food, drugs, laboratory equipment and the like. In relation to the pharmaceutical industry the relationship with the NHS can be seen to be symbiotic - more, the NHS is in effect a monopsony. This certainly gives the NHS considerable power in relation to product pricing. However, the balance of power is not entirely one-sided. Many drug companies are highly skilled in international operations, and, as the prosecution of Hoffman-La-Roche in the 1970s demonstrated, the manipulation of transfer prices can yield handsome profits. Whilst disquiet remains about some of the marketing methods and strategies employed by the pharmaceutical industry, the point is that the relationship between the pharmaceutical industry, which is entirely in the private sector, and the NHS is one of mutual interdependence rather than competition. The remorseless logic of specialisation and production costs suggests that, whilst there may be changes at the margins, little change is likely in this fundamental relationship in the foreseeable future. As an example of a 'marginal' change, there has been a gradual shift away from hospital manufacture of pharmaceutical products to private purchases of the finished article. But the question here is not about the existence of the private sector or of any drive towards privatisation but of continuing interdependence albeit with shifting boundaries. No further reference will therefore be made to this aspect of the inter-relationship.

Amenity Beds

In discussing privatisation in the NHS it will be important to isolate the influences which have led to the current debate. This is done more fully in Chapter 5 but an obvious factor in the growth of private medicine is the privacy it affords for patients. The Western Provident Association in its evidence to the Royal Commission on the NHS (1979) stated:

> 'Our experience leads us to believe that one of the principal reasons (perhaps the strongest) which leads people to subscribe to Provident Associations is to ensure the privacy of their own room when in hospital.'

The NHS has always had the means of providing privacy in what are called 'amenity' beds. There are some 3,000 amenity beds nationally (Appendix 2) and although this represents less than 1 per cent of all NHS hospital beds, the occupancy has been falling over the years. Reasons for this might include the fact that the rooms are not bookable in advance and few patients know of their existence.

Amenity beds are important not because they form any significant proportion of the total NHS complement of beds but rather because they represent a recognition by the State service of the need to provide some element of choice in accommodating hospital patients. Often there is only one amenity bed per room but sometimes two or three patients share a room. The medical and nursing care and the support services to such a patient are exactly the same as those available to a patient in an ordinary ward.

The charges in 1982 were £5.00 per day for a shared room and £10.00 per day for a single room, leading to an income for the NHS of some £280,000. Assuming that the average charge was £7.50 per day only some 37,000 patients took advantage of this facility, again an insignificant (< 1 per cent) proportion of the total deaths and discharges from NHS hospitals.

Pay Beds

Pay beds (where patients pay for their care in hospitals offering 'free' inpatient care) were first introduced in the early decades of this century in response to the rapidly rising costs of caring for patients. The increased costs were attributable, firstly, to the trend away from care at home by general practitioners towards hospital care; secondly, to advances in medical techniques and thirdly, to improvements in standards of care. The increases in costs were occurring at the same time that charitable donations, on which the voluntary hospitals mainly relied, were declining due to increased taxation. Patients in general wards also began to be asked for contributions according to a means test.

The 1948 legislation leading to the formation of the NHS embodied the principle of pay beds within the NHS and marked the acceptance by the government and the medical profession of the need for a continuing private sector of health care. The legislation also legitimised the principle of private practice within the NHS. But at that time hardly anyone could have anticipated the political battles which were to ensue about the pay bed issue. In August 1975, Barbara Castle, (then Secretary of State for Health and Social Services) produced a Consultative Document proposing the abolition of private practice within the NHS and the introduction of controls over the private medical sector to ensure that it would not extend its facilities over and above those already in existence in March 1974. The proposals generated a violent reaction from the medical profession and led to industrial action by consultants. The compromise which eventually resulted was based on Lord Goodman's formula and led to the 1976 Health Service Act, the main purpose of which was to secure the gradual withdrawal of authorisations for pay beds and facilities for private practice in NHS hospitals and to control private hospital building. The Health Services Board was set up to oversee these functions and to make recommendations for'common waiting lists' for both private and NHS patients based on medical priority alone. In retrospect it is hardly surprising that proposals to separate private practice from NHS hospitals gave a major impetus to private sector developments.

By 1977 the Board had authorised the phasing out of 1,000 pay beds and on 1 January 1980 there were 2,533 NHS pay beds left in Great Britain (2,251 in England - See Appendix 2). However, the Conservative Government had come into office in 1979 with a manifesto commitment of active support for private medicine. The commitment was translated into the 1980 Health Service Act which, amongst other things, abolished the Health Services Board and returned to the Secretary of State powers to authorise private practice within NHS hospitals. By 1982 the number of pay beds had risen by 500 to just over 3,000. The annual income for the NHS from pay beds is around £55 million but some argue that the income does not cover costs.

However, in view of the continuing controversy about the

use of NHS facilities by private patients and indeed sporadic bouts of industrial action, the Secretary of State found it necessary in 1980 to agree with the medical and dental professions a number of principles which should govern such use. The principles were designed to ensure the equitable operation of private practice in the NHS and were intended to provide additional, non-statutory safeguards for the NHS. The six principles are as follows:

(a) The provision of accommodation and services for private patients should not significantly prejudice non-paying patients.

(b) Subject to clinical considerations, earlier private consultation should not lead to earlier NHS admission or to earlier access to NHS diagnostic procedures.

(c) Common waiting lists should be used for urgent and seriously ill patients as at present and for highly specialised diagnosis and treatment. The same criteria should be used for categorising paying and non-paying patients.

(d) After admission, access by all patients to diagnostic and treatment facilities should be governed by clinical considerations. This principle does not exclude earlier access by private patients to facilities especially arranged for them if these are provided without prejudice to NHS patients and without extra expense to the NHS.

(e) Standards of clinical care and services provided by the hospital should be the same for all patients. This principle does not affect the provision on separate payment of extra amenities nor the practice of day-to-day care of private patients usually being undertaken by the consultant engaged by them.

(f) Single rooms should not be held vacant for potential private use longer than the usual time between NHS patient admissions.

Consultant Contracts

One characteristic of pay beds is that the medical care for such private patients is provided by the same consultants who care for NHS patients. The retention of pay beds in NHS hospitals means that hospital consultants can continue their private work in NHS hospitals whilst also receiving a salary from the NHS.

The Labour Party had always considered this situation inequitable and a dilution of the principles on which the NHS is based. Whilst a number of amendments have been suggested over the years, it was not until January 1980 that a new contract was agreed for NHS hospital consultants. The new Contract identifies the amount of private work permissible under the following headings:

'Full-Time' Contract -	the consultant is allowed to do a small amount of private practice but his income from it should not exceed 10 per cent of his NHS salary.
'Maximum Part-Time' Contract	the consultant foregoes 1/11th of his NHS salary in return for a slight reduction in his NHS commitments, but may undertake any amount of private practice.
'Other Part-Time' Contract	the consultant's NHS salary is pro-rata (in 1/11ths) according to his contractual commitments; he can undertake an unlimited amount of private practice.

Since the introduction of the new Contract there has been a marked shift towards 'full- time' and 'maximum part-time' contracts, in preference to 'other part-time'. At present almost 50 per cent of the 15,000 NHS consultants have full time contracts and around 35 per cent are maximum part-timers. Few consultants work entirely in the private sector. Thus, the effect of the new consultant contracts is to institutionalise the private sector within the bosom of the NHS.

Pay beds are a classic example of the intermesh between the State and independent sector, and at the same time the issue lies at the heart of the political and ideological differences of view. The differences are explored more fully in Chapter 5.

Private General Practitioners

The 1911 National Health Insurance Act was a turning point in the history of medical care in the UK. The Act instituted compulsory insurance under a contributory scheme - which provided benefits against incapacitation for work, full General Practitioner (GP) care and certain pharmaceutical benefits. One of the most important aspects of this Act was that it established the GP as the primary source of medical care rather than the hospital outpatient department.

By 1938, 90 per cent of GPs accepted patients with National Insurance, and more than a third of their income came from the Insurance Fund. Whilst constituting a major influence in defining the role of the GP, the 'per capita' payment method led directly to the referral of more patients to hospital, thus increasing the cost of hospital care, which in turn led to the increase of pay beds referred to in the previous section.

The initial proposals for the framework of the NHS in the mid 1940s drew a hostile reaction from the British Medical Association, representing both the hospital doctors and the GPs. The GPs particularly argued that being paid by salary would impose unacceptable constraints on both their personal and their professional freedom. The debate was acrimonious and prolonged and eventually Aneurin Bevan had to concede the issue of a salaried GP service in order to proceed with the major part of the principles underlying the NHS. The result was that GPs became independent contractors linked to Executive Councils (now Family Practitioner Committees) responsible for 'pay and rations'.

The position today is that more than 97 per cent of the population is registered with one of Britain's 28,000 GPs. The average size of a GP list is 2,166 although the ratio varies considerably across the country and indeed within NHS Regions and Districts. Insurance scheme statistics indicate that less than 3 per cent of the claimants consulted GPs as private patients and some of these also consulted GPs as NHS patients. The reality is that GPs who only see private patients are few in number and mostly concentrated in and around London. Although statistics are hard to come by, surveys have indicated that fewer and fewer GPs with NHS patients find the time, or find it worthwhile, to treat patients privately. There would appear to be a number of reasons for this trend:

- certain GPs indicate 'The last thing I want is the patient telling me what to do';
- the high cost of treatment; for example, a patient on multiple drug therapy with high blood pressure and a degree of arthritis could expect annual medical bills of between £100 - £200 and a drugs bill which could amount to £400 p.a.;
- few insurance companies are willing to meet these large, open-ended expenses.

A recent survey reported by the Adam Smith Institute (1982) attempted to assess whether there was substantial private demand for GP services. The survey found that with an annual subscription of about £100, some 2 million persons 'would participate immediately', with more than half the population of London expressing 'great interest once the scheme got under way'. No doubt based on the expectation of such a market for private GP care, a company called 'Medicover' was launched in 1980 to provide private home visits by GPs at any time of day or night. Subscribers paid £60 per year plus £5 per visit. The company collected £60,000 from subscribers and around £10,000 from home visits. But with the organisation employing four doctors at £15,000 each, the company traded at a loss throughout its

18 month existence and was roundly attackd by the BMA for failure to provide continuity of care. The company was 'suspended' at the end of 1981 with the 1,000 families on the books left high and dry. It is possible that this particular company encountered unforeseen commercial difficulties, but there is no evidence yet of an increase in the market for private GP care. The arguments of the proponents of this development are discussed more fully in Chapter 5.

Nursing Homes and Private Hospitals

The Nursing Homes Act 1975 requires that non-NHS institutions offering medical or nursing care to the public must be registered with the local health authority. Before the Authority can register a nursing home it must satisfy itself that the establishment meets the minimum requirements stipulated by the Act and registration is renewable annually.

A nursing home is defined in the Act as 'any premises used, or intended to be used, for the reception of, and the providing of nursing for persons suffering from any illness, injury or infirmity'. The definition leaves unclear the precise distinction between a nursing home and a private hospital. In practice, independent sector facilities range from rest and convalescent homes to ultra-modern hospitals providing the most sophisticated medical and surgical treatments in luxurious surroundings. The 1980 Health Services Act reflected this spectrum by extending the definition of the 1975 Act to include:

> 'any premises not falling within .... the preceding paragraphs which are used, or intended to be used for the provision of all or any of the following services
>
> i) the carrying out of surgical procedures under anaesthetic
> ii) the termination of pregnancies
> iii) endoscopy
> iv) haemodialysis or peritoneal dialysis'.

A crucial point of intermesh in this area is the mandatory duty on local health authorities to inspect all registered nursing homes twice a year under the requirements of the Act which specify the need for 'adequate professional, technical, ancillary and other staff'. The second major link is through staffing in that most of the senior medical input to the independent sector is provided by NHS consultants on full-time or part-time contracts. As was indicated earlier, few doctors practise entirely in the independent sector.

Thirdly, and most importantly, health authorities have been permitted since the earliest days to arrange for the care and treatment of NHS patients in facilities outside the

NHS. The original intention was that contractual arrangements with non-NHS institutions would be 'an interim measure until National Health Service Hospitals and specialist services were developed to support entirely the needs of NHS patients'. However, since 1972, contractual arrangements have been seen as an integral part of providing hospital services and in 1981, the DHSS reported that 'the use of non-NHS facilities on a contractual basis has established itself as a recognised way of providing services. Facilities used in this way have proved an invaluable supplement to local NHS institutions as an integral part of the local NHS'.

In its commitment to extending the role of the private sector, the present government has urged local health authorities to extend the range of contractual arrangements with the independent sector. The Government's thinking was embodied in DHSS Circular HC (81)1 which encouraged 'contractual arrangements with independent hospitals and nursing homes and other forms of cooperation between the NHS and the independent medical sector'.

A contract may be for an 'all-in' service that includes medical and surgical treatment as well as supporting services, or for NHS specialists and staff to use the facilities as part of their NHS contracted duties. Contractual arrangements may also be made for general practitioners to admit patients under their care.

Over the past 20 years or so, there has been a very marked reduction in the number of patients treated under contractual arrangements - both on an in- and out-patient basis - as the following table shows:

Table 3.1

Use of Contractual Arrangements in England - 1963-1980

Year	In-patient Deaths & Discharges	Outpatient Attendances	New Outpatients
1963	37,376	432,574	67,202
1965	36,569	342,361	67,084
1966	35,447	347,801	62,867
1967	34,527	360,220	63,889
1975	28,317	217,031	48,637
1976	29,046	225,991	46,625
1977	26,843	219,696	48,831
1978	26,430	191,560	49,081
1979	27,648	175,959	42,900
1980	26,705	116,530	15,857

Source: D A Horne (1982)

However, there is considerable variation between NHS Regions in the use made of contractual arrangements for clinical services. For example, South West Thames and East Anglia regions are consistently high users, accounting for 19 per cent and 15 per cent respectively of the 1980 contractual in-patient workload. In comparison, Trent and Oxford regions are low users, with 2 per cent and 1 per cent of the 1980 total. What is also interesting is that the figures confirm the generally held view that contractual arrangements are used significantly for pre-convalescent, convalescent and post-operative patients, with surgical patients constituting the second largest group.

Table 3.2

Distribution of Contractual arrangements by Specialities in England - 1980 (1979 figures)

Speciality	Inpatient Deaths and Discharges %	Outpatient Attendences %
Medicine	4 (8)	4 (3)
Surgery	18 (23)	9 (8)
Preconvalescent, Convalescent and Post operative	33 (32)	3 (1)
Geriatric Medicine	5 (5)	5 (4)
Diseases of the Chest	5 (5)	3 (2)
Maternity	3 (2)	4 (1)
Mental illness and handicap	4 (3)	4 (1)
Rehabilitation	2 (2)	11 (2)
Terminal	11 (9)	0 (0)
Others	15 (11)	57 (73)
Total	100 (100)	100 (100)

Source: D A Horne (1982)

EVEN WHEN
CONSERVATIVES
TALK RUBBISH
IT MAKES SENSE

BIRMINGHAM CONSERVATIVE COUNCIL SAVED £3,000,000 ON REFUSE COLLECTION
WIRRAL CONSERVATIVE COUNCIL SAVED £1,400,000 ON REFUSE COLLECTION
WANDSWORTH CONSERVATIVE COUNCIL SAVED £1,800,000 ON REFUSE COLLECTION
THESE ARE JUST THREE OF THE MANY CONSERVATIVE COUNCILS THAT ARE SAVING MILLIONS OF POUNDS A YEAR ON REFUSE COLLECTION

********** VOTE CONSERVATIVE **********

The above full page advertisement to the glory of privatisation first appeared in the national press on 14 May 1983 just before local government elections. But the advertisement can be interpreted in a number of ways, quite apart from the ammunition it could provide to the opposition. For example: one interpretation could be that since 1979 only a few local councils have gone 'private' - and that for one service only, refuse collection. And, indeed, local government journals carry numerous articles hotly disputing the savings claimed through privatisation.

In the NHS, whilst the debate about privatisation of non-clinical services - such as laundry , catering, cleaning, estate management - has been less public, there has been no less central pressure to 'contract out'. Appendix 3 indicates the level of contracting-out of NHS services in 1980/81. The following general conclusions emerge from the table.

Taking general services first, the gross amount contracted out was £118 million, an increase of 11 per cent in real terms over 1979/80. Contracting out was most frequent under the head of estate management, where it reached about 15 per cent of the total. Most of this was spent on buildings and engineering maintenance. Nearly 5 per cent of laundry was done on contract, mainly to supplement in-house services, or to cover their temporary withdrawal. In the case of domestic and cleaning work, 2.6 per cent was contracted out; this mainly concerned particular items such as window cleaning, though there are about a dozen large-scale hospital cleaning contracts throughout the country. Contract catering on the other hand, was negligible in 1980/81 and no portering contracts at all were reported.

More recently, Hansard for 16 March 1982 records the following information provided to the House of Commons for the financial year 1981/82:

Laundry	84 Area Health Authorities used private laundry - equivalent to 11.7 per cent of NHS expenditure on laundry services.
Cleaning	188 Area Health Authorities used commercial cleaning services - equivalent to 2.09 per cent of the NHS expenditure on cleaning services.
Catering	24 Area Health Authorities used commercial catering services - equivalent to 0.22 per cent of NHS expenditure on catering services.

The figures suggest that between 1980/81 and 1981/82, there was a decline in the proportion of expenditure on contract cleaning and catering services. The figure for laundry services in 1981/82 is not comparable with the figure for linen/laundry services in 1980/81.

In order to delve more deeply into the broad national statistics the Association of Health Service Treasurers carried out in 1981 a survey into the use of commercially provided services in the NHS. Of the 278 questionnaires sent to authorities, nearly 60 per cent were returned. The survey confirmed the broad national position that some 50 per cent of all authorities used commercial services of one sort or another with cleaning services being mentioned most often. The major reasons given for the use of commercial services were:

i) financial
ii) difficulties in recruiting staff
iii) inability to provide facilities themselves

The survey also revealed that most authorities seem to be satisfied with their existing arrangements primarily because their main difficulties (e.g. staff recruitment and retention, trained supervision, administrative problems, or cost/benefit exercises) had been resolved with the employment of the contract firms. Most authorities had no current intention of extending their use more widely, but would probably continue their existing contractual basis when it came up for renewal. An important finding was that although there had been savings on costs in some instances, costs were generally only of equal importance with the other problems of staffing, supervision and administration. The conclusion of the survey was that there was little purpose in a national move towards commercialisation because this did not offer a universal panacea for greater economy or efficiency; but that in some circumstances a local initiative in this respect could solve local problems.

The government's recent exhortations are designed to persuade local health authorities to contract-out clinical and non clinical services on a much wider scale. How a particular district is responding to these pressures is set out in Chapter 6. However, it is important first to consider the relative sizes of the public and private sectors of health care in order to put the debate into context and the next Chapter undertakes this comparative analysis.

4 Origins, size and growth of the health care industry

Historical Perspective

This is not the place for a detailed historical analysis of the origins of the NHS or of the independent medical sector. Nevertheless, an understanding of the present complex nature of the 'industry' requires a brief examination of its antecedents.

For the majority of people in the nineteenth century personal health care was virtually non-existent. The poor had, in effect, only two sources of medical care available to them - the infirmary attached to the local workhouse or a voluntary hospital if one had been established in the area in which they lived. Workhouse infirmaries were considered a last resort by most people. Administered under the Poor Law of 1834 by Boards of Guardians - generally lay people - the aim was to save rate-payers money. Conditions in these infirmaries were harsh and medical attention often very limited.

Voluntary hospitals were monastic in origin and many were founded during the 18th century by philanthropic laymen for the benefit of the sick poor. They grew considerably in numbers during the 19th century and, as they were often staffed by well-qualified surgeons and physicians who gave their time free, these voluntary hospitals gradually developed into centres for research and teaching. The wealthy usually received their medical attention at home or in their physician's consulting rooms, as hospitals could be very dangerous places until the early 20th century when control of infection became a reality.

The first major change of the 20th century to affect the relationship between the doctors, the state and the community was occasioned by the National Health Insurance Act of 1911. As was indicated earlier, the Act, whilst having little direct effect on voluntary hospitals, had considerable long term repercussions in that the role of the GP as the first point of contact and as the main referral agent to hospitals became the norm. By 1929 the groundswell of opinion against the stigmatising effects of the previous practice (the 'workhouse' syndrome) led to legislation which in turn led to an increase in the provision of municipal hospitals. These public hospitals, which also included the old infirmaries, provided some 75 per cent of hospital beds during the 1930s. They were financed mainly from local rates and block grants from central government. Patients were charged according to means, unless they were out-patients or suffering from an infectious disease. All staff were paid - salary for full-time doctors and sessional fees for part-time consultants.

During the 1930s, co-operation between the public and the voluntary hospitals grew, with a broad division of labour emerging - the public hospitals taking many chronic, infectious and maternity cases, while the voluntary hospitals took the more acute and short term cases.

The onset of the war led to the establishment of the Emergency Medical Service and the Emergency Hospital Scheme, and by the 1940s it became clear that a large scale reorganisation of existing health services would be desirable. Following widespread consultation, the then Minister of Health, Earnest Brown, announced in 1941 the decision to create a National Health Service after the war. A major influence on the debate about the shape of a future NHS was the report published in 1942 by Sir William Beveridge ('Social Insurance and Allied Services') which put the health service in the context of the wider question of social security. In 1944, a White Paper was published on a National Health Service, the primary objectives of which would be that 'in future

i) every man, woman and child can rely on getting all the advice, treatment and care which they may need in matters of personal health;

ii) that what they get shall be the best medical and other facilities available;

iii) that their getting these shall not depend on whether they can pay for them, or on any other factor irrelevant to the real need - the real need being to bring the country's full resources to bear upon reducing ill health and promoting good health in all its citizens'.

The original concept was that only the municipal and Poor Law hospitals, together with those voluntary hospitals so choosing, would be grouped together under the control of Local Authority Joint Boards. In addition, State financing and control was to be geared towards <u>basic</u> medical care. By the time the NHS came into being on 5 July 1948, Aneurin Bevan, the generally acknowledged 'father' and 'midwife' to the NHS, was able to include all voluntary, municipal and Poor Law hospitals within the NHS. The role of the NHS had also changed from providing <u>basic</u> services to providing a <u>comprehensive</u> service 'free at the time of need'. The National Health Service Act 1948 embodied what was hoped for:

Sec 5.1 (i) 'it shall be the duty of the Minister to promote the establishment of a comprehensive health service designed to secure improvement in the physical and mental health of the people and the prevention and diagnosis and treatment of illness, and for this purpose to provide or secure the effective provision of services in accordance with the provisions of the Act.

(ii) The services so provided shall be free of charge except where any provision of this Act expressly provides for receiving of charges'.

At this time there was widespread acknowledgement of the poor state of the nations's health but also the belief that the cost of the new NHS would decline, or at least remain stable, as the pool of unmet need was gradually removed. In retrospect, this was one of the most serious misconceptions in the grand strategy. The table below indicates how the costs of the NHS have increased over time.

Table 4.1
Growth of NHS Expenditure

Year	Total Exp £m	Total NHS Exp as % of GDP	Total NHS Exp per head of popn	Total NHS costs at 1949 prices £000
1949	437	3.92	8.74	437
1959	826	3.84	15.88	545
1969	1797	4.48	32.52	839
1977	6919	5.45	123.99	1220
1978	7861	5.39	140.79	1280
1980	11875	6.14	212.04	1445
1981	13524	5.91	241.50	1481

Notes: 1. GDP at factor cost

Source: Compendium of Health Statistics 1981 published by Office of Health Economics.

Despite the more than three-fold increase in real terms in NHS resources there is a widespread view that the NHS has failed. It may be that the rumours of the death of the NHS have been exaggerated, but there is little doubt that the UK spends proportionally less than other western countries on health care, as the table below illustrates:

Table 4.2
Health Care Expenditure on all Services (public and private) as a percentage of GNP

Year	Australia	Canada	France	West Germany	Italy	Netherlands	Sweden	Switzerland	United Kingdom	United States
1950		4.0	3.4				3.4		3.9	4.5
1955		4.3	4.5			4.0	4.1		3.4	4.4
1960	5.0	5.6	4.7			4.5	4.7		3.8	5.3
1965	5.2	6.1	5.8		5.0	5.3	5.6	3.8	3.9	6.2
1970	5.5	7.1	6.4	6.4	6.1	6.3	7.4		4.3	7.6
1975	7.0	7.1	7.9	9.4	7.1	8.1	8.5	6.9	5.5	8.6
1977	7.9	7.1	7.9	9.2	6.4	8.2	9.8	6.9	5.2	8.9
1978	8.0		8.2	9.2					5.2	8.9
1979			8.4						5.2	9.0
1980									5.6	9.4

Source: Maxwell (1981)

The NHS now employs more than 1 million people. Some key statistics relating to the services provided are set out in the following table:

Table 4.3
Key NHS Statistics

No of hospitals (1980)	2,501	declining
Staffed beds (1980)	440,900	declining
Average daily occupation (1980)	355,400	declining
No of deaths & discharges (1980)	6,808,000	increasing
No of hospital medical staff (1980)	28,235	increasing
No of hospital dental staff (1980)	1,220	little change
No of hospital nursing staff (1979)	299,139	increasing
No of midwifery nurses (1979)	20,149	including pupils
Community nursing staff (1979)	32,162	increasing
No of general medical practitioners (1980)	28,413	including trainees
No of general dental practitioners (1980)	14,316	including assistants

Source: Various DHSS Publications

Some 89 per cent of NHS expenditure is financed from the Consolidated Fund, with National Health Insurance contributing about 9 per cent and Charges about 2 per cent. The proponents of private medicine argue that since the public purse is finite, encouraging private health care is a way of increasing the resources going into health care. This view is explored more fully in Chapter 5.

Independent Sector - Size and Growth

Table 4.2 indicates the share of the national cake devoted to health care. The relative proportions of the public and private sectors is more difficult to assess, but the table below provides a broad indication of the split.

Table 4.4
Expenditure on Health Care as % of GDP (mid-seventies)

	Private %	Public %	Total %
Britain	0.6	4.6	5.2
Germany	1.5	5.2	6.7
France	1.6	5.3	6.9
Sweden	0.6	6.7	7.3
United States	4.3	3.0	7.4

Source: 'OECD' (1977)

Turning now to the size of the independent sector, the scale of facilities has changed as follows in recent years. (Table 4.5 includes all premises whether called 'nursing homes', or 'clinics' or 'private hospitals', registered or licensed under appropriate legislation.)

Table 4.5
Independent Sector Facilities

Year	No of Units	Aggregate bed capacity	Average beds/unit
1975	1,217	29,551	24.3
1976	1,220	32,103	26.3
1977	1,217	32,403	26.6
1978	1,278	33,376	27.2
1979	1,221	33,556	27.5
1980	1,229	34,404	38.0
1982	1,265	35,628	28.2

Source: Registered Nursing Home Association: Reference Book (1982/83)

The table illustrates that whilst the number of units remained steady up to 1980, the aggregate bed capacity has gradually increased, leading to a higher average number of beds per unit. However, 1982 shows an increase both in the number of units and in beds and, although not certain, it is likely that the present government's policies are now being reflected in the growth of the private sector. There has also been an increase in the deaths and discharges from independent hospitals and nursing homes as follows:

1978 - 157,177

1979 - 167,093

It is estimated that some 170 of the units in the above table are acute hospital units providing about 6,500 beds. Since the mid 70s, this is the sector which has examined fastest and it is estimated that another 800 beds are planned and a similar number are under construction.

Basic accommodation charges in the independent acute hospitals can vary from about £120 per day to over £200 per day in the most luxurious commercially operated hospitals. In practice, many of the luxury class hospitals tend to cater specifically for foreign patients and, in some, such patients account for more than 75 per cent of the total occupancy. Over and above the basic charge, private patients are liable to pay for drugs, dressings, theatre fees, surgeons' fees, etc.

Private Health Insurance - Historical Development

In many ways the scale of private sector operations is judged better by looking at the insurance scene rather than merely at facilities. Here again, it is helpful to provide a brief historical perspective to appreciate the present context of private care.

Historically, the voluntary hospitals were financed mainly by voluntary payments from those who could afford to make some contribution towards the cost of their accommodation and treatment and partly by charitable sources of revenue. After the middle of the 19th century they also enjoyed a growing source of income through associations with contributory schemes of pre-insurance under which working men in employment clubbed together to provide for treatment in sickness by small weekly payments in times of good health. The role of these 'Friendly Societies' changed little during the early part of this century except that many of these and the Provident Clubs became linked with particular hospitals, giving contributors a moral, if not legal, right to treatment as in-patients or out-patients.

In the 1920s there was a growing awareness that, due to high taxation and inflation, there was a need for some type of health insurance scheme geared to the requirements of the lower income groups. In 1922, the Hospital Savings Association (HSA) was founded. The scheme provided for free hospital care in the general wards of voluntary hospitals in return for 3 pence a week or 12 shillings for a year.

The first serious attempt to meet the needs of the middle income patient was the formation in 1923 of the British

Provident Association. Unlike the HSA scheme, there was no income limit and the annual subscription was one guinea.

During the inter-war decades the British Provident Association expanded gradually whilst a number of other provident associations also came into being during this time. With the coming of the NHS, these associations came under severe threat given the expectation that few people would be prepared to pay premiums to insure against fees for private treatment on top of the compulsory National Insurance contributions which would entitle them to free treatment in the public wards. Faced with this threat to their existence, most of the provident funds decided to form a united national association and the British United Provident Association (BUPA) came formally into being on 3 April 1947.

Present Size and Future Growth

Over the years since 1947, three associations have dominated the private health insurance market. The three are BUPA, the former London Association now operating as Private Patients Plan (PPP), and the Bristol scheme which has retained its identity and now operates as the Western Provident Association (WPA). These three associations account for 98 per cent of the total subscription income, with the breakdown as follows:

BUPA	71%	of total subscription income
PPP	23%	" " " "
WPA	4%	" " " "

There are also six small associations with long established local ties in Bristol, Exeter, Bedford, Norwich, as well as associations linked to the Civil Service and the Inland Revenue. These smaller associations have steadily held some 2 per cent of the subscription income i.e. they too have grown with the larger associations. Table 4.6 below identifies the rate of change over recent years:

Table 4.6
BUPA, PPP, WPA - Subscriber Trends

Annual Rate of Change (+)

Period	No of Subscribers	Subscriptions Earned	Benefits Incurred
1956/61	9.6%	17.9%	17.7%
1961/66	7.8%	15.4%	16.1%
1966/67	6.0%	17.5%	16.2%
1971/76	1.6%	24.2%	22.3%
1976/77	0.0%	28.6%	21.7%
1977/78	5.8%	15.8%	4.6%
1978/79	15.6%	16.2%	24.1%
1979/80	27.5%	26.4%	52.0%

Source: Lee Donaldson Associates (1980)

By the end of 1981, the three major associations covered about 4.1 million people, of which 3.0 million were covered by BUPA. In that year, these three associations had a combined subscription income of £203m and paid out some £196m in benefits. Since the end of 1978 the provident population has increased by about 1.4 million persons. The rapid growth in the last few years was preceded by years of mixed fortunes. During the 1950s and 1960s, the provident population showed steady and persistent growth. The position changed in the mid 1970s when for the first time growth slackened and in 1975 and 1976 the provident population fell. After these two slack years growth was restored in 1977 with a rapidly rising trend to produce the recent record increases. Subscription income has tripled since 1975 with benefit payments following a similar pattern although lagging a year or two behind substantial growth of subscription income. Appendix 4 sets out some of the key statistics over the period 1955 to 1980 and Appendix 5 highlights key points from the 1981 Reports and Accounts of the major health insurance schemes.

It is of course very significant that some 7.5 per cent of the national population is now covered by private health insurance. But the pattern of subscription is also revealing. Subscribers may join the provident associations under a variety of different schemes. The traditional form, which dominated the provident population during the early years, was individual membership. During the 1960s, there were developments, first of schemes promoted for company employees, and then of schemes aimed at individual members of professional and trade bodies. The table below shows that the number of individuals enrolling rose throughout the 1960s, then declined until 1978 and then has risen rapidly.

Over the same period, the more rapid growth was concentrated in either the occupational or in-company group schemes, the latter showing the sharpest increase.

Table 4.7
BUPA, PPP, WPA - Subscriber Numbers

Year	Individual Schemes	Occupational Schemes	Company Groups	Total
1964	264		368	632
1965	277		403	680
1966	292		443	735
1967	304		480	784
1968	314		517	831
1969	325		561	886
1970	328		602	930
1971	334		652	986
1972	328		693	1,021
1973	324		740	1,064
1974	312		784	1,096
1975	294	361	432	1,087
1976	275	335	447	1,057
1977	257	320	480	1,057
1978	249	317	552	1,118
1979	257	333	702	1,292
1980	267	510	870	1,647

Source: Lee Donaldson Associates (1980)

The growth in the number of subscribers has been reflected in rises in the number of claims and the number of private patient episodes, as table 4.8 illustrates*

* The term episode refers to the number of times a patient utilises a health care service.

Table 4.8
BUPA, PPP, WPA - Indices of private patient claims and estimates of episodes

Year	Claims		Private Patient Episodes	
	Indices 1971 = 100	Rates per 000 insured	Number (000s)	Rates/000 insured
1971	100	206	n.a.	n.a.
1972	94.2	188	n.a.	n.a.
1973	96.8	185	n.a.	n.a.
1974	106.2	197	130	56
1975	111.3	209	132	57
1976	115.9	223	139	62
1977	120.1	231	134	59
1978	122.2	222	142	59
1979	135.5	213	160	58
1980	177.2	215	212	59

Source: Lee Donaldson Associates (1980)

However, the rates per thousand insured have not changed significantly over the period, leading to the conclusion that subscribers make use of the private facilities at a more or less constant rate. The mix of hospital treatment has, however, shifted gradually over time with major operations (46 per cent in 1980 claims value) declining slowly and intermediate and minor operations showing a slight increase. The major item of expenditure is accommodation and nursing charges (about 51 per cent) followed by surgeon's fees (26 per cent), and other specialist fees (2 per cent).

Before leaving the question of insurance funds, it is important to mention for completeness two other areas. Firstly, there are now emerging commercial carriers of private health insurance - Crusader Insurance Co Ltd and Allied Medical Assurance Services Ltd are amongst the first in this field. Both organisations concentrate on company schemes and their health care premium income amounts to between 1 per cent and 2 per cent of the total attracted by the Provident Association.

Secondly, Hospital Contributory Schemes (HCS) provide cash benefits in case of illness irrespective of whether the treatment is private or under the NHS. Their traditional aim has been to help meet higher domestic costs associated with illness and in recent years they have increased the scope of cover to meet contributors' NHS charges. These schemes are in decline as table 4.9 shows.

Table 4.9
Hospital Contributory Schemes

Year	Contributors (000s)	Persons Covered (000s)	Premium Income £000	Benefits Paid £000
1974	3,346	8,365	10.96	8.38
1975	3,295	8,237	12.61	9.71
1976	3,297	8,242	15.45	11.56
1977	3,151	7,877	17.57	13.31
1978	3,176	7,940	19.93	14.63
1979	3,100	7,750	23.11	16.68
1980	3,005	7,512	27.46	20.48

Source: Lee Donaldson Associates (1980)

Whilst there is no denying the rapid increases in private health insurance, all is not peace and harmony within the independent sector of medicine as might be supposed. The following is an extract from the Chairman's statement in the 1981 BUPA annual report and typifies current tensions in this sector.

> 'Our growth rate, particularly in the present economic climate, continues to be satisfactory, although inevitably it was much lower than in the previous year, when there was what we all knew to be a wholly exceptional increase. It is unfortunate that some commentators chose to regard that year as typical and to base upon it forecasts of the future demand for private medicine that were totally unrealistic, even going so far as to assert that by 1985 some 12 million people, nearly one quarter of the population, would be privately insured.
>
> 'This exaggeration has had three disturbing results. First, it has encouraged a small, local and unrepresentative minority who as a matter of political dogma are opposed to independent medicine, to claim that the private acute sector was now competing unfairly with the NHS for scarce resources, particularly for nurses. In fact, as against the NHS establishment in England alone of about 190,000 qualified nurses, there are in the private acute hospitals in the whole of the UK, only an estimated 7,000 and this figure is almost equalled by the number of 5,673 who were registered as unemployed at the end of the year.
>
> 'Secondly, commercial insurers, mostly from abroad, have begun to move in to what they seem to have believed was a very large and rapidly expanding

market. Some are doing so by quoting what appear to be loss-making premiums unlikely to be maintainable after the initial business has been secured, especially against the background of similar difficult conditions in their own markets.

'Thirdly, private developers have begun to plan and build hospitals on a substantial scale. There are clear dangers both that some areas may become over-bedded and that the profit motive can lead to excessive charges, not always for beds, but sometimes for drugs and other services. Where this has happened, it has inevitably led to higher benefits being claimed by our subscribers and this in turn has put pressure on our subscription rates. It is not surprising that some of our large subscriber groups have become so concerned about this that they have begun to advise their employees not to use such hospitals where reasonable priced alternative facilities of high standard are available.

'Escalating costs are becoming a major problem of independent medicine ....'

The private developers to whom the Chairman referred are mainly large corporations which have grown rapidly over the last decade in the USA and are now attacking overseas markets in a concerted way. Amongst these darlings of the American Stock Exchanges are American Medical, Humana Corporation Inc and Hospital Corporation of America. At the last count, American Medical had six hospitals in operation and two under construction, Humana had three in operation and three under construction and the Hospital Corporation of America had launched a vigorous drive for a share of this market.

Although in contrast to the network of hospitals operated by non profit making organisations, such as the Nuffield Nursing Homes Trust (a charity established and mainly funded by BUPA), the profit making sector is yet small but its impact on the scene has been dramatic. The above statement by BUPA's Chairman referred to the escalation of costs and the statement can be described as diplomatic. In fact, there is little love lost between the two sub sectors within the independent sector, even though one depends heavily on the other for its existence.

Independent hospitals, a number of which are in the Greater London conurbation, rely heavily on private patients insured with the provident funds - some two thirds of private acute hospital patients are covered by private health insurance - but during the 1970s a significant proportion of their trade came from the highly priced 'inelastic' Arab trade. Of late, this trade has dwindled somewhat as the oil money is used to build the most sophisticated acute hospitals in the Arab homelands. As indicated in the BUPA Chairman's statement the home market may not be able to bear the prices previously charged and demand might therefore dwindle. Indeed, the relationship between the two sub sectors reached its lowest ebb when a well publicised national symposium on the independent medical sector to be held during 1982 had to be cancelled because the provident associations refused to share the platform with speakers from the profit making sector.

An even more recent development has been the failure of American Medical's most recent and technologically advanced hospital, the Chaucer Hospital in Kent, to attract the anticipated in-patient demand. In March 1982, the press carried reports that a number of the nurses were being made redundant and that the capacity formerly reserved for in-patient care was being adapted to provide day care for which there is thought to be greater demand. This publicity reinforces the views of those opposed to private medicine who argue that market forces should not be the only determinant in the provision of health care and are particularly hostile to the international corporation which, it is suggested, has little regard for continuity of services or employment. This point is further developed in the next Chapter.

5 Arguments for and against private medicine

The Protagonists

Apart from the health care institutions themselves, the main participants in the national debate on privatisation in health care are the political parties and the Trade Unions. Health care is one of the issues where it has become the norm not to practise what one preaches - namely that health care is too important an issue to be treated as a political football. It may be that during the 1960s there was a political consensus about the role of the NHS. Alas, any such consensus has long since evaporated. In retrospect, it would have been naive to expect that the issue would remain non political, no matter the convenient slogans.

Having accepted that health care is inevitably of major political significance it also becomes evident that the distance between the main political parties is now greater than perhaps it has ever been, particularly since any discussion of the independent sector is incomplete without taking into account the implications for the NHS.

The battle lines are drawn. The Conservative Party in the shape of the present government is committed to an expansion of the private sector. The Labour Party is completely opposed - its manifesto for the 1983 General Election reaffirmed its commitment to the NHS, to the removal of private practice from the NHS and indeed the nationalisation of parts of the independent sector. The Trade Unions also have a large vested interest - NALGO has 90,000 members in the NHS, COHSE has 213,000 and NUPE has over 300,000.

Insofar as the postures of the protagonists are underpinned by philosophical, economic or social beliefs it is important to consider what arguments are marshalled for and against private medicine. This Chapter sets out these arguments and shows that many of the points are closely interlinked, for example the issues about freedom of choice, the quality and quantity of services, cost and efficiency and industrial relations.

The Question of Choice

One of the main arguments (in its simplest form) of those in favour of private medicine is that a service provided only by the State restricts individual choice. The argument goes that those who wish to spend their money on private health care should have the option of doing so since they already contribute towards the cost of the NHS. In ideological terms, this argument takes the form of the principle that private medicine is good precisely because it conforms to the spirit of free enterprise. In its extreme form, the argument reflects a hankering for a return perhaps to the free market 'paradise' of the nineteenth century. The present system, it is claimed, is dominated by the State and provides no mechanism for consumers to express their preferences. Those who so argue, advocate the introduction of competition in health care. Jacques (1976) distinguishes between two types of competition - 'service providing' compeitition and 'labour exploitive' competition. In relation to the first he says:

> 'Service providing' competition is manifestly in the interest of society. It is socially bonding in the sense that availability of choice gives a sense of freedom to consumers, as against the paranoigenic restrictionism of a monopolistic situation, whether private or public. Moreover, competition of this kind requires those accountable for bureaucratic work and its output of goods and services to orientate themselves to understanding and fulfilling the human needs they are supposed to be satisfying.
>
> It is in connection with this last point that competition emerges as one requisite feature of bureaucratic functioning. One of the main reasons for the development of the pejorative meaning of bureaucracy as red tape bound monoliths is connected with those bureaucratic systems in which any possibility of competition from other bureaucratic systems is legally precluded as, for example, in the case of most government departments and social services. In the absence of competition, it is easy for standards to fall; or conversely, it is difficult for standards to rise.'

The main counter argument to this is generally that the experience before 1948 demonstrates that free market forces have failed to provide adequate and appropriate health care. A whole battery of statistics can be marshalled in support of this contention. For example, it is evident that the doctor/patient ratio is highest in London and other large cities and significantly lower in rural and economically depressed areas. Morbidity and mortality rates are correlated with occupational and economic classifications - the poorer you are, the more you are likely to be ill and the less access you have to health care facilities and services. In a free market, it would be natural for health care resources to be attracted to those areas which yield an economic rate of return, rather than to respond to notions of equity, or egalitarianism.

Whilst the arguments above have been put in their starkest form and few now argue openly for the dismantling of the NHS, privatisation is thought by its opponents as being an insidious process and all the more dangerous for that.

Quality and Range of Services

Linked closely to the question of choice is the argument that the independent sector of medicine should be enlarged because it provides a higher quality of care which can only be to the advantage of the community. This argument begs the question - What does the patient get, or hope to get, from having his operation performed privately that he feels he will not get as an NHS patient? Since most of the patients in Britain are entitled to free treatment, having contributed towards the cost of the NHS, they must have expectations that make them willing to pay all over again.

The first reason usually given is that the operation will be carried out by a surgeon of the patient's choice who has a personal contractual relationship with him - the question of choice again. On closer examination it is not easy to sustain this claim. The vast majority of consultants who operate privately are in fact NHS consultants. The channel for either private or NHS referral to a consultant is generally through a general practitioner. Whilst it is true that general practitioners have usually developed special links with particular consultants, few general practitioners would in reality turn down a request from a patient for referral to a named consultant. The contractual relationship between the consultant and the patient is certainly no different whether the patient is a private one or is treated as an NHS patient.

The second quality of care argument certainly holds more water. This is that the operation can be performed to suit the patient's convenience. Convenience may have two aspects - access to treatment quickly and access to treatment at a time convenient for the patient. In relation to the first aspect, there is little doubt that delays in admission to NHS hospitals can be unacceptably long depending on the locality and the speciality.

A private hospital is often able to accommodate patients sooner than an NHS hospital. However, there have in the past been fierce controversies regarding the earlier admission of private patients to NHS pay beds which led to Section 6 of the Health Service Act 1976, requiring arrangements to ensure that 'all persons admitted or afforded access to accommodation or services in NHS hospitals as resident or non resident patients are, so far as practicable, admitted or afforded access thereto on the basis of medical priority alone, whether they come as private patients or not'. This Section was inspired by the widespread belief that private patients obtain priority of treatment in NHS hospitals over NHS patients. The Health Services' Board, which examined this issue (1977), did not accept that admissions to hospitals were governed by 'medical priority' alone and pointed out that doctors also took into account the following factors, depending on the individual's circumstances:

1 pain and discomfort suffered by the patient,
2 the length of time the patient has been seeking in-patient admission,
3 the patient's domestic circumstances including his dependency on community support services (for example, the effect his housing might have on his condition),
4 the patient's occupational circumstances (for example, teachers seeking admission during school holidays),
5 the patient's willingness or ability to enter hospital at the time offered,
6 the availability of hospital diagnostic and treatment facilities,
7 the availability of hospital staff,
8 the need to balance admissions for major and minor conditions to ensure practical operating lists and balanced nursing workloads,
9 the need to admit patients with a variety of conditions to assist professional teaching and training (particularly in teaching hospitals).

The Board went on to recommend that 'all patients (other than emergencies who were handled in the same way in any case) should be placed on the same waiting list as comparable NHS patients in the care of the same consultant'.

Whilst these recommendations went some way towards taking the heat out of the highly emotive issue of 'queue jumping', the reality of long waiting lists and long waiting times remains in the NHS. As at August 1982, some 720,000 people in England were awaiting admission to NHS hospitals. The question, therefore, has to be asked -'Can the NHS be improved to the point where patients no longer consider it worthwhile to pay private medical insurance?' The answer is likely to vary depending on the viewpoint of the commentator. One view is that only a lack of resources is preventing the NHS from overcoming its known difficulties. In the extreme, this view says that for ideological reasons there is a deliberate ploy to starve the NHS of resources so as to create a supply vaccuum which the private sector can fill. This is in effect the 'thin edge of the wedge' argument. Others argue that the demand for health care is always likely to outstrip supply and this process will be accelerated by the new technological advances in medicine, leading to the frustration of the rising expectations of the population.

The truth, as usual, perhaps lies some way between these

two viewpoints. There is no doubt that the founders of the NHS fundamentally miscalculated the nature of demand for health care - hence, the 'clearing of the backlog' expectation which was prevalent in the 1940s. On the other hand, there is little doubt that some of the greatest inadequacies in health care provision can only be attributed to a lack of resources and could be remedied.

A third argument in relation to quality of care is that private medicine allows care to be provided in circumstances that are pleasant, private and can be modified to suit the patient's personal needs. There is perhaps more than a ring of truth in this implied criticism of public sector medicine. Certainly, when medical circumstances demand, NHS patients can, for example, be accommodated in single rooms. Nor is the quality of service generally low - indeed, by international comparisons, NHS staff are some of the most skilled and dedicated in the world. Nevertheless, the NHS is, in reality, a small number of huge organisations, which inevitably suffer from the inadequacies and inflexibilities of a national sponsored bureaucracy. There is much in the literature on the subject of behaviour in organisations which could be usefully applied to dealing with 'customers' in NHS hospitals, particularly to overcome the impersonality of large public hospitals. There has, in fact, already been a backlash from the 'big is beautiful' concept of the 1960s towards smaller hospitals with their focus on the local community. But much remains to be done to achieve the level of personal attention which is claimed for private hospitals. Additional resources will no doubt help, but perhaps the major emphasis needs to be on the development of the attitudes which encourage courtesy and consideration, not only for the client, but also for relatives. A typical example of this is where relatives are telephoned to reassure them at the end of a major operation.

But even those who argue for the extension of private practice recognise that it has an unacceptable face, although they go on to describe this as an 'abuse' rather than as a major feature of this sector. Opponents are quick to point to the experience of private sector medicine in the country often held up as the haven of free enterprise - the USA. Even a senior member of the present government recognised the heavy 'human cost' of the unacceptable face when a former Secretary of State warned the US Pharmaceutical Association in 1977:

> 'Ten million Americans lack any private or public insurance to pay for health care and many more have inadequate cover. In 1970, ill health accounted for a third of all personal bankruptcies. Market forces are pretty ineffective in balancing the need for health care and the supply of services.'

In the United States it is now widely recognised that a

consequence of commercial medicine has been the increased use of high cost technology, of services which are inappropriate, irrelevant and unnecessary. A classical example was the race by American hospitals to acquire the whole body scanner since hospitals not having this equipment felt in danger of losing 'customers' to those that did, even though the diagnostic power of the equipment was appropriate in but a small proportion of cases. An American anaesthetist, Bunker (1974) has shown that the USA has twice as many operations per person as England and Wales at all age levels. The difference is mainly acccounted for by 'discretionary' operations suggesting the American practice that, if it pays well to circumcise, remove gall bladders, intestines etc, then ' whip it out'. Another statistic indicates that if you live in the USA you are 20 times more likely to have your appendix removed than in the UK.

There would appear to be three main reasons for this over-use of expensive technology and procedures under commercial systems. The first, and probably the most important, is the fee per-item-of-service method of payment to doctors by insurance companies rather than, as in the NHS, salaries, capitation payments and systems that reward judgement. In a health insurance system, doctors largely generate the demand for their own service. In the words of Professor Abel-Smith (1976), one of the most respected authorities on health care systems:

> 'The highest financial rewards go not to the best doctor, but to the quickest, and to the doctor with the least professional scruples about responding to the financial incentives of the payment system. Some doctors may even claim for services which are not performed.'

The second reason has already been mentioned, namely the need in a competitive environment for product differentiation in the form of the most modern equipment, whether necessary for treatment or not. Finally, the fear of prosecution for negligence may fuel the necessity to order costly investigations and tests, not because they are really needed but to cover against malpractice suits. Almost 10,000 malpractice claims against doctors are filed each year in the USA.

An important aspect of the argument about quality and range of services is that related to the view that in the absence of rationing by price, rationing has been by inconvenience, unavailability and queueing. For example, it is said that demand for the service of general practitioners has led to a reduction in the time available for consultation and an increase in the time spent awaiting consultation. A 1966 study had over half of its doctors reporting that more than 25 per cent of their consultations were for 'trivial, unnecessary or inappropriate reasons'. A

1974 study found that 28 per cent of consultations were not for medical services at all. Of those who did come for treatment, some 43 per cent showed no definite illness. There can be little doubt that faced with increasing demands and severely curtailed resources, the waiting list is a form of rationing. Enoch Powell (1975), a former Minister of Health, has suggested that :

> 'the worst kind of rationing is that which is unacknowledged, for it is the essence of a good rationing system to be intelligent and consciously applied. This is not possible in the NHS where its very existence has to be repudiated.'

In one sense, the waiting list is helpful to ensure that the expensive consultant facilities are fully utilised, but present waiting lists exceed this minimum requirement for the full employment of the medical resources. But whether a larger private sector will have any effect on NHS waiting lists is discussed more fully in Chapter 6.

Questions of Cost and Efficiency

Reference has already been made at a number of points to the cost and financial arguments for and against privatisation. The following sections look at a number of facets of this question.

The pro-privatisation lobby argues that at a time of increasing financial stringency one way to increase the resources available for health care is to encourage non-governmental sources of finance. A number of methods are suggested for stimulating this additional flow of funds, most of which rely on instituting measures to encourage the demand for private health care. One method which this present government has already implemented is allowing tax relief on private health insurance premiums for employees earning less than £8,500 per year. This, it is argued, should be extended by removing the earnings limit.

The argument goes on to suggest that two effects could be expected as people opt out of the public sector - a decrease in pressure on public sector services and at the same time an inflow of funds to the private sector from non-governmental sources.

It must be said that these arguments are based on economic theory rather than on hard evidence. There is, for example, little evidence that those who make use of the private sector will no longer use the NHS. This is illustrated clearly later in this section. And, unless a substantial proportion of the population does opt out of the NHS, the pressure on the NHS is unlikely to decrease because of the unique relationship of supply and demand identified earlier. Demand has historically far outstripped supply and this is likely to continue since the NHS will then be able to undertake many of the things which it is presently unable to do - the classic dilemma of supply creating its own demand.

A related point is that, whilst there is a general view that market forces lead to greater efficiency than is possible in the public sector, this phenomenon may not hold up so well in the health care industry. For example, administration costs of the NHS could no doubt be reduced, but at less than 5 per cent of 'turnover' compare favourably with the following (Klein 1980):

Belgium	12%
France	12%
Australia	18%
USA	21% - 30% (estimates vary).

These countries have a much higher proportion of their health care costs funded through private health insurance. And the reality is that the administrative and financial task of selling insurance packages, and the examination and payment of doctors' bills acording to a fee schedule, is expensive. Germany, for example, has 1,600 individual health insurance funds which require 80,000 staff to operate them. There is little dispute that the marginal costs of raising funds through private health insurance are significantly greater than the cost of those raised through general taxation.

However, opponents of private medicine argue an even more potent economic case - potent because it uncovers some of the insidious effects of drifting into private medicine. The argument begins from the reality that the taxpayer does not in fact pay for most of the care he receives from the NHS. During the period of his life when he pays most taxes, our national average man is on the lowest point of his lifetime use of the NHS. It is the old and, to a lesser extent, children who place the heaviest demands on the NHS. During the 1970s, the 65-75 age group used three times as much of NHS resources, per head, as the 16-64 age group. The imbalance is even greater above age 75, with six times the expenditure per head of the working age group. Thus, the taxpayer finances not his own care but that of the elderly. The chart below illustrates some of the relativities in per capita costs at different ages.

Table 5.1
NATIONAL HEALTH SERVICE - ANNUAL COSTS PER PERSON: BY AGE AND SEX, 1979 - GREAT BRITAIN, £ PER PERSON

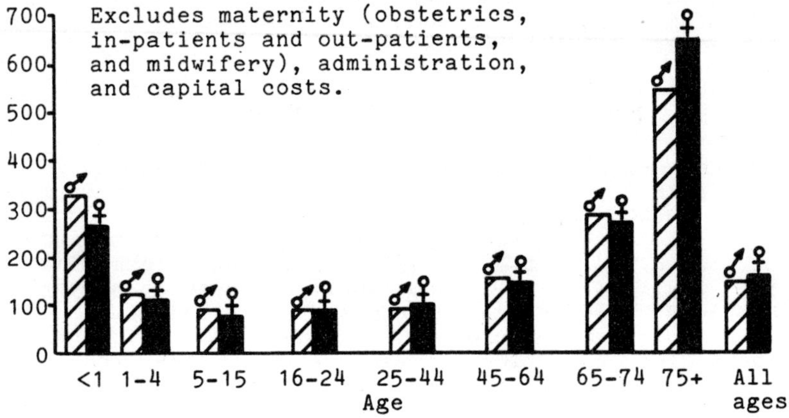

Source: Central Statistical Office

On the other hand, the inequality of use of the service by different age groups is, of course, central to private insurance. It is precisely because the population of working age uses health services so little that it is possible for private health insurance to be so relatively cheap - the premium for a family being of the order of a packet of cigarettes per day. Similarly, the need for care and its costs are so high among the over 75s that insurance has little point and would carry a premium very close to the cost of care. Where then is the threat to public health services? As mentioned earlier, surely if those with private care continue paying taxes but take their demands elsewhere, then the elderly would benefit? Obviously they would, but is it plausible that the growing numbers with private cover will continue to be enthusiastic supporters of political manifestos pledged to raising taxes and improving the NHS? People are likely to be reluctant to pay for a service never received, little realising that they may be all too grateful for it in old age. Resources for the care of the elderly will dwindle if this happens - and a system separating old from young will develop.

Many people now covered by private insurance will inevitably drop into the NHS in old age. Much of private cover is met by employers and so will end at retirement age, a time of falling personal income and rising premiums. The private insurance companies are generally unable to offer to take premiums now for care in 30 years' time, since the cost of safeguarding against rising costs and inflation would make the premiums wholly uncompetitive in the market place. In the end, it is the State which will have to meet the costs of caring for the aged. Ironically, say the opponents, the danger of private insurance is that it will encourage those who wish to shed the moral burden of taxation, not out of meanness, but out of a failure to appreciate who the NHS really serves.

Employee Relations

One of the most pervasive fears of Trade Unions in the NHS is what privatisation might do for the employment prospects of their members. This is so mainly for manual workers - some 80,000 full time equivalents in England employed in domestic cleaning services, 24,000 in portering and 29,000 in catering. It has traditionally been argued that, like the Civil Service,, NHS employees have enjoyed almost complete protection against the cold winds of the competitive market place. In addition, it is argued, the terms and conditions of service are better than in many sections of the wealth-creating sector of the economy.

Privatisation would affect employment and employees in the NHS in a number of ways. The most obvious case is where a service presently provided in-house is to be contracted out to a private company. The immediate reality is redundancy for some, if not all, because the private contractor claims to be more efficient precisely because he can provide the same level of service with fewer staff. Even if some of the existing NHS staff are re-employed by the contractor, it is highly unlikely that the terms and conditions of service would be comparable - for example, the emotive issue of index linked pensions. There is also the fear that , where jobs are not lost, privatisation will drastically reduce the career prospects of NHS employees.

The opponents of private medicine argue that the difference between the NHS and private enterprise is the difference between the managers on the spot. This discrepancy exists, it is suggested, because the NHS has neglected the middle managers who are consequently underpaid and undertrained. Rectifying these two deficiencies, it is claimed, would go a long way to making up for any productivity gap. Further, it is argued that directly employed staff also provide the intangible but valuable benefits of loyalty and experience.

A related argument is that the private sector 'creams off' scarce staff trained at national expense. For example, all nurses and doctors are presently trained in the public sector. Recognising the truth of some of these allegations, the private sector is attempting to make some efforts towards training its own staff. Some companies in the private sector have been discussing with the General Nursing Council the possibility of recognition of private hospitals for training purposes. An even more interesting proposal is from a consortium which proposes to purchase the recently vacated Royal Free Hospital Medical School in order to open a private medical school to be known as the Hunter School of Medicine. The school is intended to offer a five year degree course at £6,500 a year and is expected to take in about 50 undergraduates. The school would award degrees of the independent University of Buckingham. It will be interesting to see whether this venture will be accepted by the various professional organisations and whether the graduates of the school have the same standing as those from the State system.

The survey conducted by the Association of Health Service Treasurers mentioned earlier (1981) also included discussions with full time union officials. The opposition of the Unions to privatisation was stated by the officials to be for the following reasons:

1 there is evidence that standards are reduced;
2 despite promises to the contrary, rates of pay and conditions of service are not protected;
3 cleaners and other ancillary staff are an integral part of ward teams and the therapeutic community of hospitals. Outside firms cannot provide this integrated teamwork with other professions;
4 NHS organisations lose control of costs, standards and efficiency of commercial services. Payment by results is no substitute for true and involved management;
5 time and resources have been devoted to the training and development of senior officers, supervisors and foremen/women in all categories. This would be wasted. In fact, the Unions indicate that the outside firms 'cash in' on the training in which the NHS has invested;
6 and the Unions know that many organisations (both within and outside the NHS) have had to revert to direct provision of services after unfavourable experiences with contract cleaners etc. These major changes and staff movements have been against the interests of the NHS, the patients and staff involved.

But the Trade Unions are no longer united in their opposition to privatisation in health care. Some unions not represented in the health service have already accepted free private health insurance as part of the remuneration package. The Amalgamated Union of Engineering Workers, and the NUT are two of these and the latest addition to this list was a Civil Service Union. The initial stance of the Royal College of Nursing was that they had no objection to the development of the independent medical sector so long as the comprehensive coverage of the NHS was not undermined. However, the body wished to see pay beds taken out of the NHS. Over recent years this stance has become modified somewhat and, although it would not wish pay beds to be integral with NHS beds, it suggests that they should be in close proximity. Doctors for their part are thought to be wholly in support of private medicine, but there are some factions which would not wish to see the NHS threatened by a large private sector - the NHS Consultants Association is one such group. NALGO has mounted a £1m publicity campaign entitled 'Put People First', against privatisation in local government and the NHS, NUPE and COHSE are not far behind. Appendix 6 sets out the resolution passed at the 1982 NALGO annual conference regarding private medicine. These three unions cover a significant proportion of the non clinical staff in the NHS and therefore continue to represent a substantial opposition to privatisation in health care.

This Chapter has concentrated on the many arguments for and against the development and growth of the private sector of medicine. These general arguments are certainly in evidence within the NHS at local level and local health authorities will need to take account of them in responding to local privatisation initiatives. The next Chapter briefly outlines the structure of the NHS, which is an important factor in how new threats and initiatives are tackled, and then considers a series of case studies relating to privatisation in one local health authority.

6 Case studies in privatisation

Chapter 1 emphasised that the approach taken in this monograph has been a pragmatic one focussed on how the NHS might cope with the concept of privatisation. Chapter 2 went on to identify the different ways in which the process of privatisation is intended to operate. All these methods affect the NHS as an organisation, but the most direct and evident is where the NHS is being required by the government to change the way in which it operates so as to advance the concept of privatisation.

This Chapter sets out how the government has attempted to bring influence to bear on the NHS and how the organisation has responded. The material for this Chapter is taken from the events in one local health authority - District X. This initial examination of organisational processes is followed by 5 'Case Studies' which set out the way in which the District has attempted to respond to the pressure to privatise and the many complex organisational and practical issues which the attempt has raised.

Structure and Process

The NHS is a 'public' service precisely because the Secretary of State for Social Security is accountable to Parliament for its operation. However, to enable him to discharge this accountability, he relies on the Department of Health and Social Security for policy advice and on the fourteen Regional Health Authorities (RHAs) and 190 District Health Authorities (DHAs) for the strategic planning and operational management of the service (Fig 6.1). The DHSS, being a central government department, is staffed by career civil servants - but only 5,000 of the 30,000 employees of the department work within the health service section.

The chairmen and members of RHAs are appointed by the Secretary of State following wide local consultation and appointments are intended to bring a wide cross section of expertise and skill to the management and planning of the health service. At District level only the chairman of a DHA is appointed by the Secretary of State, all the other members being appointed by the Regional Health Authority. The RHAs are responsible to the Secretary of State for the discharge of their responsibilities, and DHAs are responsible to RHAs. Whilst an authority can technically be stripped of its powers if it fails in its duties, this is an extremely rare occurrence. Usually, the interaction is one of influence and persuasion on both sides. Thus it is that

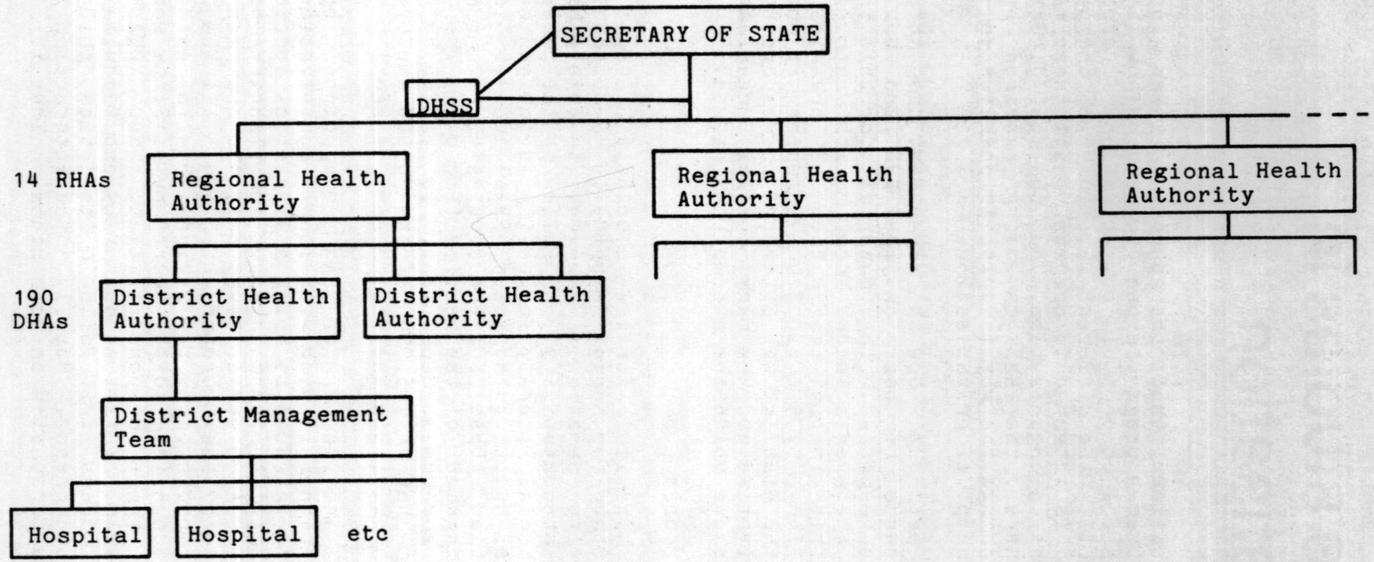

Figure 6.1 NHS Organisation Chart

the Secretary of State provides 'guidelines' on how the health authorities should spend the money allocated to them and the steps they should take to effect the Government's policies. The sheer magnitude of the task has prevented Ministers in the past from monitoring 'performance' in other than the broadest terms. However, things may be changing. During 1982, the Minister instituted a process of review whereby the Secretary of State holds a meeting with each RHA and asks the RHA to explain in considerable detail its achievements over the past year and its targets for the future. RHAs in turn are expected to undertake the same process with their DHAs. With only one cycle complete, it is difficult to say how this mechanism will evolve but clearly it can be a powerful tool to hold health authorities to account for the way in which they pursue Government policies. The present structure came into being in April 1982.

The thrust towards privatisation in the NHS began soon after the election of the present Government in 1979. Initially, the activity was restricted to Ministers extolling the virtues of the independent sector of medicine with general expressions of hope that the NHS would seek additional ways of collaborating with the private sector and that the private sector would seize opportunities coming their way and grow in size. In a letter to chairmen of health authorities in June 1979, the then Minister of Health announced a number of steps to allow the Government's manifesto commitments to be achieved;

- restoration of the Secretary of State's discretion to allow NHS hospital facilities to be made available for private patients, to be achieved partly by the abolition of the Health Services Board;

- mechanisms for making it easier for private hospital development to proceed without challenge from the NHS up to a specified limit beyond which the Secretary of State reserved the power to make authorisation;

- encouragement for a fresh approach to cooperation between the NHS and the private sector, including the possible increased use of contractual arrangements;

- possibilities for sharing of some staff and perhaps collaboration in research.

The Government's initiatives on private medicine were launched at a time of considerable turbulence and uncertainty within the NHS. The Royal Commission on the NHS had published its report in July 1979 and there was a general expectation that the NHS would be reorganised yet again. The Government's proposals on restructuring were first announced in early 1980 and began the very considerable organisational task of removing one tier from the management structure and appointing and staffing to a new structure. At the same time, the economic recession had eaten into the developement resources available to the NHS and there were widespread fears of large scale cutbacks in services. The response of the NHS to the Government's initiatives on private medicine, therefore, need to be seen in the light of the other preoccupations of the NHS.

The success of any Government initiative can only be judged in so far as it affects the scene at the local level. The following sections set out the way in which one health authority - called District X here - responded to the initiatives. It must be said that there are wide variations in the demographic, resource and management characteristics of districts and the following is in no way a 'typical' response. Neither are the 'Case Studies' a statement of good or bad administrative practice. Nevertheless, the 'Case Studies' assist in identifying a number of policy issues with which the NHS needs to grapple if it is to ensure that the objectives for which it was established are not subverted - and at worst that it does not become the provider of 'second class services to second class citizens'.

CASE STUDY 1:

Amenity Beds

In 1981/82, District X had 'notionally' available 68 amenity beds, representing 1.7 per cent of the District's total bed complement. Of these, 50 beds are in a small hospital for the mentally ill and only 18 beds are in acute and general hospitals. However, the 68 amenity beds yielded an income of only £3,840 in 1981/82, showing that, at best, the occupancy was just 3 per cent in terms of bed days.

During the same year DHSS took a number of steps to encourage health authorities to increase the provision and use of amenity beds:

- previous requirements for central authorisation of amenity beds were removed and health authorities were allowed to establish as many beds as appropriate

- health authorities were encouraged to publicise the availability of such beds to patients prior to admission and to make the necessary administrative arrangements to meet requests for amenity beds.

The local response to this central initiative was mixed. Whilst concurring with the objective of meeting patients' needs for privacy, the District identified a number of practical difficulties. The first was indeed recognised in the original legislation which said that amenity beds could only be provided if the single room or small ward was not required by another patient for medical or nursing reasons. Reflecting this, the relevant information booklet issued to prospective in-patients in the District said that whilst amenity beds were available it was 'probable' that the patient's request might not be met. Secondly, it was suggested that in the older hospitals there were few opportunities for creating single bedrooms or small wards. Thirdly, if demand outstripped supply, a separate waiting list would need to be kept causing administrative difficulty. In addition, the admission of the patient might have to be unduly delayed in order that the request for an amenity bed could be met. Fourthly, it was suggested that the physical separation of amenity beds would increase the work of nursing staff who are already fully stretched. Finally, it was suggested that publicising the amenity bed facility would lead to frustration since the request would often have to be refused.

At the conclusion of the debate within the District, the wording in the patient information booklet was slightly amended to make it sound less discouraging for those who wished to use an amenity bed. There would appear to have been litle change in demand for amenity beds and indeed the pressure remains to reduce the number of such beds drastically in view of the low occupancy.

CASE STUDY 2:

Pay Beds

The Health Services Board was abolished with the passing of the Health Services Act 1980. In effect, the Act gave the Secretary of State power to authorise the establishment of pay beds in NHS hospitals provided that 'market demand for such facilities could be demonstrated' and, in contorted legislative phraseology, 'subject to the requirement ..... that the authorisation and use of such accommodation and services should not to a significant extent either interfere with the performance of any duty imposed under the 1977 Act to provide accommodation or services to the disadvantage of persons afforded admission or access to health services accommodation otherwise than as private patients'.

At the time of the Act, District X had a 'group authorisation' of 20 pay beds. This meant that whilst there were in fact 36 beds designated as private beds, not more than 20 could be in use at any one time. Of these designated pay beds, 30 were in the 'pay bed wing' of one of the general hospitals of the District, an old building which does have single rooms but which cannot compare in fixtures, fittings and facilities with the standard of the private hospitals now being built. Nevertheless, a number of NHS consultants undertook private practice at the unit and in fact there were many occasions when demand for beds meant that patients had to be discharged earlier than desirable in order to keep to the 'group authorisation' of 20 beds. In 1981/82, the District had an income of £800,500 from private resident patients and a further £66,000 from private non resident patients (i.e. day patients, out-patients etc). The charges for pay beds are of the order of £100/day for a single room and the patient pays medical fees directly to the consultant. Charges are also made for any X-ray or pathology services used.

At about the time of the 1980 Act, the first phase of a large new teaching hospital was being completed in the District. It was clear that the hospital would attract highly skilled staff but also patients from a wider catchment than usual, partly because of the prestige it was likely to acquire and partly because of its major medical teaching responsibilities. A number of NHS consultants who work at the hospital saw the obvious opportunity to undertake private work at the hospital and submitted a detailed case to the Authority for the establishment of 11 pay beds at the hospital. These beds were to be additional to the designated 36 pay beds already in existence and the request was that the 'group authorisation' be increased from 20 to 30 beds. The Authority, before reaching a decision, consulted widely on the proposals. The unions were formally consulted but neither they nor other management and professional groups made many substantial comments. The local private sector objected strongly, seeing the proposals as an obvious threat to their business objectives. The consumer watchdog, the Community Health Council, agreed to the proposals provided that the 'six principles' of private practice in NHS hospitals identified in a previous section were followed. The proposals were subsequently submitted to the Secretary of State who gave the necessary authorisations. No analysis has yet been undertaken of how the additional beds are functioning in relation to the demand for private care in the District.

CASE STUDY 3:

Contractual Arrangements - Clinical Services

Appendix 4 sets out the extent of contracting out by the NHS in England in 1980/81. In relation to clinical services, £45 million was spent on outside contracts in England in 1980/81; £18 million of this was on maintenance of technical equipment, and the remaining £27 million on contractual arrangements with the independent sector for the use of about 3,000 of their beds. Most bought-in hospital care is for elderly and mentally ill people. Also, the voluntary sector fills an important gap in the provision of sterilisation and abortion services, and private sector diagnostic equipment, such as head and body scanners, have been used by the NHS.

Reference has already been made to the way in which Ministers declared their commitment to privatisation following the election of the Conservative Government in 1979. One of the first concrete steps the Secretary of State took in relation to the NHS was the publication of Circular HC (81) 1 on ways in which the NHS could enter into contractual arrangements with the independent sector of medicine for the treatment of NHS patients. The circular identified three potential areas where contractual arrangements might be used:

- short term use to overcome temporary difficulties in provision of NHS services e.g. to tackle long waiting lists or to maintain a level of services while NHS facilities are closed for building work;

- medium term contracts e.g. before new capital facilities become available;

- long term contracts enabling more effective use of total resources.

On receiving the circular, District X undertook an assessment, necessarily for the first time, of the scale of the private medical sector in its midst. It was found that there were some 13 independent sector establishments providing 372 beds, and proposals existed for an increase in the size of one establishment by 22 beds and the setting up of a new private hospital with 70 acute medicine beds. Most of the establishments contained only medical beds, often providing nursing care for the elderly, but three establishments also provided surgical beds and facilities. The circular removed any administrative or legal bars to the District entering into contractual arrangements with any of these private operators and indeed a number of local and national private hospital operators contacted the District offering contractual arrangements for a variety of clinical services. Appendix 7 is part of an advertisement for one such establishment which contacted District X.

The District next looked at its own services to determine what scope there might be for contractual arrangements. It came to the view that there was little doubt that waiting lists were unacceptably long in some specialities and, what is more important, the wait before admission was also unacceptably long as tables 6.1 and 6.2 below illustrate:

Table 6.1

URGENT CASES: waiting time at 30 September 1980

Speciality	Cases who had already waited over 1 month	Total Urgent Cases	%	Rank Order by %
General Surgery	93	115	81	3
Geriatrics	80	94	85	2
Orthopaedic Surgery	4	6	67	5
Gynaecology	116	209	79	4
Plastic Surgery	161	164	98	1

Source: See Footnote*

Table 6.2

ROUTINE CASES: waiting times at 30 September 1980

Speciality	Cases who had already waited over 1 year	Total Non-urgent cases	%	Rank Order by %
General Surgery	270	1226	22	7
ENT	929	2341	46	4
Orthopaedic Surgery	1061	2938	36	5
Gynaecology	1035	3231	32	6
Dental Surgery	52	108	48	3
Plastic Surgery	1272	1706	75	2
Mental Handicap	132	154	86	(1)

Note: Urgent cases should be admitted within one month at the latest. Routine cases should be admitted within one year at the latest.

Source: See Footnote*

---

* Footnote: The tables and the issues identified in this Case Study are taken from a document prepared by District X for internal discussion. Although the data is now some years old, the issues arising for privatisation remain valid for other acute specialities.

Plastic surgery emerged as a speciality with difficulties in both tables. The District was already aware of this but because of a shortage of operating theatres, the deficiency was unlikely to be rectified for a number of years. There appeared little prospect that the District could recruit an additional consultant who could in turn reduce waiting lists and waiting time. Thus, in terms of the Circular, plastic surgery offered the potential for contractual arrangements both in the short and the medium term.

However, further discussion within the District revealed a number of obstacles to proceeding with contractual arrangements with the independent sector:

1 Balance of Investment

The allocation of additional resources to plastic surgery would inevitably mean that improvements in other services would have to be deferred since the District, like the NHS as a whole, worked to cash limits. Both nationally and locally, priority has been given to improving the 'Cinderella' services - namely those for the elderly, the mentally ill and the mentally handicapped - whilst expenditure on acute services was to grow at a slower pace. The District's pattern of expenditure was already skewed in favour of acute services and the proportions would be skewed further as the new acute teaching hospital was opened. There was, therefore, a conflict between the need to meet immediate pressures and the achievement of the District's strategic objectives.

2 Demand and Supply

There was in any event evidence to suggest that waiting lists once reduced by special means such as contractual arrangements for an agreed number of cases may not stay at the lower level permanently. One reason for this may be that the criteria for getting on the NHS waiting list becomes easier. The implication is that contractual arrangements for a specific number of cases may not be successful in reducing the waiting lists permanently. Again, since NHS workload and costs do not reduce, lower waiting lists and waiting times can only be obtained by a permanent increase of services, either within the NHS or outside it.

3 Inter-Organisational Relations

The danger exists that the use of contractual arrangements may serve to deflect the responsibility for providing care for the priority groups e.g. elderly etc from those other agencies statutorily charged with providing such care. To take one example, services for the elderly in the District are substantially below the desired level. Part of the difficulty is that some patients occupying hospital beds should more appropriately be cared for in sheltered housing or Part III accommodation*, the responsibility of District Councils and the County Council respectively. The placement of geriatric NHS patients within the independent sector may lead to a spurious reduction in the pressure on hospital beds and hence the influence which health authorities have on local authorities to fulfil their statutory responsibilities. Even more fundamentally, resources diverted to contractual arrangements may reduce the pace of developments in the domiciliary and community services for the elderly, developments which are regarded nationally and locally as helping to provide a better quality of life for the individual and allowing more appropriate use of hospital facilities. Incidentally, it is to be noted that inappropriate or inadequate levels of NHS service might itself distort the training arrangements for the NHS professions.

4 Questions of Cost

The DHSS circular had said that authorities should give early consideration to contractual arrangements where they allow 'the best and most economical provision of services'.

In 2 above, entitled Demand and Supply, it was concluded that contractual arrangements are likely to constitute a net additional cost to the NHS, and indeed a net recurrent cost if the arrangements are to have a permanent impact on the provision of services. The other side of the coin is that the development of the independent sector may in turn reduce or indeed eliminate the use of pay beds within the District's hospitals which yields nearly £900,000 per annum to District X.

5 Relative Costs

The more specific question of whether a particular service is cheaper to provide within the NHS or through contractual arrangements is more difficult to answer because the accounting systems in the NHS do not allow each case in each speciality to be costed precisely. However, some general points can be made in regard to relative costs. It is relevant to note that the NHS carries essential overheads which the independent sector does not. One example of this is the costs incurred in training the whole range of health service staff, and particularly medical and nursing staff. Since some 70 per cent of the NHS budget is comprised of staff costs, the costs per case in the NHS may well be

---

* Part III refers to the duty of local authorities to provide accommodation to those in need of care and attention under Part III of the National Assistance Act 1948.

higher, for example, in a geriatric hospital than in a private nursing home. However, since the overheads remain unchanged and occupancy in geriatric hospitals is high, the marginal cost of admitting a patient to a geriatric ward may well be lower than the charge levied by an independent nursing home, based on their average costs.

6 Capital Costs

One other very important point in relation to costs is that the NHS treats capital as a 'free good'. Any real comparison of costs will, therefore, require agreed conventions on how to include the cost of capital in the calculations.

7 Clinical and Legal Responsibility

Circular HC (81) 1 says at one point:

> 'Health authorities have overall responsibility under the NHS Act 1977 for providing treatment on the part of an organisation providing services on its behalf under contractual arrangements. Authorities should therefore consider providing in the written contract that the contractual establishment take out necessary insurance cover and indemnify the authority against any damages it was made to pay in respect of the negligence of the establishment's staff'.

The above makes clear that in proceeding with contractual arrangements, health authorities will be required to play a very much more substantial role in relation to the independent sector than is required under the Registration of Nursing Homes Act 1975. The task of drawing up contracts, of monitoring standards, selecting and channelling patients to the contractor are tasks in which health authorities have little experience and which will place a heavy demand on administrative time and medical and nursing resources at a time when the Government has made much of its intention to reduce administrative staff and costs on a substantial scale. For example, the Minister of Health at that time claimed that the administrative restructuring in 1982 would save £30 million.

In the face of the above points, the District concluded that,

> 'there are neither the resources nor obvious service reasons for undertaking a comprehensive review of existing provision to identify opportunities for entering into contractual arrangements. Indeed, the timing of such a review in the context of the forthcoming restructuring of the Health Service is inappropriate'.

Instead, the District noted

> 'that Circular HC (81)1 highlights the potential for entering into contractual arrangements as another option that can be considered for solving problems in service provision and for planning the future pattern of services now that the administrative and statutory bars to such arrangements have been lifted'.

CASE STUDY 4:

The Family Planning Case

Following the above conclusion, the District would have been content to let matters lie until a more opportune time. It was not to be. A number of members of the Health Authority became increasingly anxious that the budget for family planning procedures was being continually and substantially overspent. Family planning in hospitals is one of the few cases where consultants and pathologists are paid on an item-of-service basis, in addition to their salaries. In other words, the Health Authority faced an open ended commitment to meet the fees of all the family planning procedures the consultants chose to undertake. Faced with severe resource constraints, the problem for the Health Authority was one of persuading the consultants to keep within budgets. But a subtler element was concern within the medical community itself that some of its members were able to earn substantial sums in addition to their salaries. It was also argued that family planning procedures were displacing more essential work.

At the same time as the above debate was taking place within the Authority, a local private establishment, called Forest Grange here, wrote to the Authority offering to undertake family planning procedures at stated rates, with discounts if significant numbers of cases could be channelled their way. The dilemma for the Authority was, firstly, lack of experience in undertaking contractual arrangements and, secondly, arriving at comparative costs on which to base a judgement. But more importantly, the difficulty was to negotiate with the NHS consultants a limit to the number of remunerable cases they could undertake, an extremely sensitive issue, if family planning costs were to be contained within the total available budget.

The initial response of the District was to receive the offer from Forest Grange for future action. However, the proprietor of the establishment was extremely persistent and the Authority, therefore, undertook a cost comparison exercise. The results of the comparison in their entirety are set out in Table 6.3. The following comments can be made about the costing exercise.

1 Because of the way in which the accounts are kept in the NHS, it is extremely difficult to put precise costs to an in-patient stay. Therefore, the line on 'other direct costs' is an average based on 3 different ways of calculating such costs.

2 For laparoscopic sterilisations, the cost for a volume contractual arrangement appears significantly cheaper in overall cost terms but not in terms of direct costs. However, NHS resources would be released for other procedures (which in turn will generate further costs).

Table 6.3
Financial Comparison for Family Planning Procedures NHS Vs Forest Grange

Procedure 1: Laparoscopic sterilisation under General Anaesthetic

(a) NHS Costs

Direct Costs

Blood tests (2)	£2	(estimate)
Clinician's Fee	£45	
Anaesthetist's Fee	£22	
Other Direct Costs	£10	(estimate)
	£79	
Indirect Costs associated with 24 hour stay	£66	(estimated)
Estimated total NHS Costs	£145	

(b) Forest Grange Offer

Operation including blood tests	£65
General Anaesthetic	£10
Overnight Stay	£75
	£150
Discretionary Discount on overnight stay for volume	(60)
Total: Forest Grange Costs	£90

Procedure 2: Vasectomy (under local anaesthetic)

(a) NHS Costs

Direct Costs

Clinician's Fee	£33
Pathologist's Fee	£12
Other Direct Costs	£02
	£47
Indirect Costs	£05 (estimate)
Estimated Total NHS Costs	£52

(b) Forest Grange Offer £35

3 For vasectomy, a contractual arrangment appears cheaper in terms of both overall and direct costs. NHS resources would also be released for other procedures.

The results of the cost comparison were put into a paper for consultation with medical staff who would have to agree if the contract was to be arranged. The process of consultation has been so extensive and the issue so sensitive, that a correspondence begun during 1981 had not been concluded at the time of writing (June 1983). The proprietor of the establishment has alleged that the Authority has been dilatory in reaching a contractual arrangement with his establishment and has written to his Member of Parliament.

CASE STUDY 5:

Contractual Arrangements - Non Clinical Services

Whilst in relation to clinical services the first major national initiative was in the shape of Circular HC(81)1, the initiative in relation to non clinical services took a slightly different form. In fact, the then Minister of Health wrote to the chairmen of all health authorities urging them to consider 'contracting out' in a range of non clinical services. The letter, which is attached in full at Appendix 8, required a reply and in District X stimulated the first formal review of existing and possible contractual arrangements. The reply which was eventually despatched to the Minister made the following points:-

1 Supplies. One firm had approached the District offering a specialist service to provide commercial sterile packs. The firm however had since closed its local factory. Another firm was offering a laundry and linen service and this offer would be kept in mind should changes be contemplated to the current satisfactory arrangements.

2 Transport and Vehicle Maintenance. The District had a contract with a local firm for a motor cycle despatch service; short term hire of vehicles was also undertaken; the vehicle and ambulance fleet was maintained by the local authority but this arrangement was to be reviewed.

3 Pharmaceutical Services. All products, except for non injectible sterile water, were purchased commercially; special formulations required by medical staff could only be produced in-house.

4 Works Services. The general policy was to maintain approximately a 60/40 balance of work between the use of contractors and the use of direct labour; certain tasks could only be undertaken by direct labour e.g. wall washing in operating theatres at night.

In conclusion, the Chairman's reply said: 'All our arrangements are kept under continuous review, and our District Works, Supplies and Pharmaceutical Officers are very conscious of the economic need to be constantly aware of the spirit of your letter.'

Whether the reply satisfied the Minister is not known. But commercial organisations were not slow to react to the potential profitability of the massive £2,216 million market for NHS general services. District X received approaches from a wide range of companies offering a variety of services. Not the least aggressive of them were companies in the cleaning, laundry and catering industries, the Trade Associations of which had been discussing opportunities with the Minister of Health. Faced with this barrage of offers, the District could do little but respond to say that the offer was noted until such time as administrative time was available to undertake the necessary comparative work.

But a start had to be made somewhere and the District began by holding exploratory discussions with four contract cleaning companies. The report submitted on the discussions concluded that only two of the four companies were of sufficient size to be capable of providing contract domestic services to a large hospital. Both these companies had been keen to emphasise that they had resources and expertise amassed over several decades in this field and were not 'fly by night' operators. No financial comparisons were undertaken but the report ended with a summary (Appendix 9) of the case for and against the employment of 'hotel services' contractors in the NHS.

Even as these preliminary conclusions were being assimilated by management in District X, the DHSS issued in February 1983 a draft circular on 'NHS Support Services - Contracting Out'. This large package of paper amounted to some 140 closely typed pages and contained the following:

- a policy statement on the use of the private sector;

- Appendix 1 to the statement setting out the procedures to be followed where a health authority sets out to test the cost effectiveness of existing services by going to tender;

- Appendix 2, which is a model tender and contract for the provision of domestic services to the NHS;

- Appendix 3, which is a model tender and contract for catering services;

- Appendix 4, which is a model tender and contract for commercial laundry services;

- Appendix 5, which is a model tender and contract for commercial linen and garment rental services;

- Appendix 6, which gives the addresses of the Trade Associations for the relevant services.

This detailed document with major implications for the NHS was published on 22 February 1983 and comments were invited by 31 March 1983 - during a time when the NHS was deeply involved in the upheaval of organisational restructuring.

The first two paragraphs of the policy statement said:-

> 'The Government believes that the use of commercial contractors, under carefully drawn and properly controlled contracts, can often prove the most cost effective way of providing hospital support services. It is, therefore, right that health authorities should seek tenders from outside contractors and from their in-house service on a basis of fair comparison.
>
> 'The Government's expenditure plans envisage that growth in the health services will in part depend on efficiency savings. The need for efficiency applies of course to all services, but the scope for savings in domestic, catering and laundry services is potentially high, and authorities need to be wholly satisfied and to demonstrate that those services are

provided as efficiently and economically as possible'.

On receiving the 'carefully drawn' model contracts, District X sought legal advice. The solicitor's response was:-

'The model form of contracts are so far removed from what could be regarded as satisfactory, that my strong advice to the health authority would be that no contract should be let on the basis of the models until I have had the opportunity to consider them in more detail and draft amendments which are appropriate to safeguard the interests of the authority'.

In replying to the contents of the draft circular the District added a whole range of other caveats:

1 the circular did not appear to recognise that Trade Unions might not wish to cooperate in the move towards privatisation. In this event the NHS could be confronted with major industrial relations problems.

2 there was doubt that in many cases local industry would have the capacity to cope with the demands placed on it; in any event, there was the danger of 'monopoly' arising from handing over critical services to the only firm in the area;

3 the arrangements suggested did not recognise the safeguards essential in services provided by outsiders in close proximity to patients;

4 the circular made no mention of the significant staffing and cost implications of tendering and supervision of contracts.

And there the matter rests at the time of writing. District X has concluded that the approach to contracting out requires a 'cautious but positive' approach and thought is being given to the possibility of experimenting with a cleaning contract for a small hospital unit. However, the matter may not be as simple as that. NUPE, which was represented at the Authority's discussions on the subject, subsequently wrote a letter, some key paragraphs of which are as follows:

'(to) the Government's policy to provide the most cost effective support services, my comment would be that I believe the facts of the matter are that the Government are pursuing a political ideological approach.

With reference to the Government Plans for future

NHS growth depending on efficiency savings, we feel that the District should protest on this matter, particularly as the Government has already shown a lack of commitment to NHS growth.

'I have to say that bearing in mind the statements made by Government Ministers and the ideology of this Government, the staff will have many fears because they will feel that fair comparisons will not be made. Indeed, we are aware of such things as loss leaders, and questions of accountability. The information already available to the union from the experiences encountered by local authorities would seem to show that in many cases contractors seek to introduce unfair competition with a view to winning the contract, thus destroying the infra-structure of the direct labour service, bringing about a monopoly situation in which they are able to dictate the terms of future contractual arrangements'.

7 Towards collaboration at the local level

A Proactive Approach

About three years ago the Royal Commission on the NHS concluded its review of the independent sector of medicine by saying:

> 'The difference in scale of the private and public health care sector suggests that private practice could have, at most, a marginal and local effect on the NHS ..... it is clear that the private sector is too small to make a significant impact on the NHS, except locally and temporarily'.

The previous Chapters indicate very clearly that the conclusion of the Royal Commission would now be an unacceptably complacent response for a health district given the rate at which the private sector has expanded and is continuing to expand.

By implication, there would no longer appear to be room for continuing to ignore the private sector in the hope that it is the product of a particularly 'free market' orientated government and that another government of a different complexion would remove any threats the NHS faces. As a matter of financial reality no government would have the resources necessary to nationalise the private sector of health care and thus hand over private hospitals to the NHS. More fundamentally, whilst election manifestos may continue to carry an ideological flavour, there would appear to be in practice much evidence to suggest popular disenchantment with monolithic, monopolitic public enterprises which are seen as a charge on economic prosperity. Indeed, there is a widespread view that the growth of public spending on welfare programmes is a prime cause of economic decline. If, then, the private sector is here to stay, the NHS at local level has little alternative but to move away from the present uneasy form of co-existence to a more thoughtful appraisal of how to manage the changing boundaries between the sectors.

The argument for a District to adopt a more pro-active stance has both a defensive and a positive side. On the one hand the NHS at the local level needs to guard against the danger that a random growth of the private sector might undermine the very principles which appear to have wide acceptance - for example, the principle of equality of access to health care. On the other, there may indeed be possibilities for the NHS to use the private sector in ways which allow the District's objectives to be achieved.

Privacy

However, before turning to this issue it is as well to recognise that the growth in the private sector is partly an expression of the dissatisfaction with some of the services provided by the NHS, or at least the manner in which these services are provided. Reference was made in an earlier Chapter to the danger that a service such as the NHS can become 'producer orientated' rather than 'consumer orientated' and there is a range of lessons which the NHS could learn from the private sector. For example, an organisation with the management skills of the NHS and dedication to patient care should not find need to quote 'administrative difficulties' in justifying the low priority it has given to meeting patients' needs for privacy, particularly since the provision of amenity beds could generate a small but useful income. Surely, it should be possible to gain a true measurement of demand for such a facility by actually making it easier for patients to ask for and be given such a facility. Nor is there justification for suggesting that management time is required for issues of greater import - this claim could indeed be true in terms of the strategic objectives of the NHS but paradoxically may undermine those very objectives if individual patients leave NHS care feeling they have been 'processed' by an impersonal State machine. In a similar way, it should not be difficult to recognise that, in addition to the undoubted dedication medical and nursing staff bring to the care of an individual patient, there is the important task of ensuring that the patient's relatives are given appropriate reassurance and support. This has been in the past not a failure of dedication to the caring and curing task but of a narrow interpretation of the needs of patients and relatives. It may be added that such a service does not require the latest facilities and staffing comparable to that in private hospitals - but rather the more general application of good patient care practices which already exist in many parts of the NHS.

Pay Beds

Although there has been some increase in the number of pay beds (about 500 beds nationally) following the removal of restrictions by the 1980 Act, the growth has been relatively small for the reasons identified earlier. In District X for example, only 11 additional pay beds have been established since 1980. There can be little doubt that in strategic terms, pay beds will decrease in importance as the independent sector grows. Thus, there is little to be gained by a District in taking any initiatives on its own account but rather to recognise the income which they generate, and their value as a means of retaining the goodwill of senior medical staff. The task is mainly to respond if the local medical staff wish, and are able, to make a case for additional beds. Perhaps an additional task would be to make further improvements in pay bed facilities but this would generally be a highly political issue and in any case not possible in many Districts, given the constraints of existing old buildings. It may well be that provident associations could be persuaded to make donations to finance the upgrading of NHS private patient facilities for the benefit of their members generally. Alternatively, the suggestion of the Royal College of Nursing, that pay beds should be separate from, but close to, NHS could be extended to allow the management of these beds to be handed over to the independent sector.

Gathering Intelligence

Returning to the question of collaboration with the independent sector, it was suggested above that the NHS at local level needs to be proactive in its approach. In order that more considered policies can be adopted, it is vital that a District assemble the necessary information about the independent sector in its midst. This may not be as easy as it sounds, as the gathering of information for this study has demonstrated. Unlike the NHS, the independent sector does not adopt a common format for the information it collects and distributes and therefore a number of channels will need to be pursued. Clearly, some basic information is already available to Districts through the procedure established for the Registration of Nursing Homes. But in order to get a comprehensive picture of the local scene, recourse may need to be made to direct contact with each establishment; closer liaison with the local authority to establish plans for adaptations, extensions and new hospital developments; examination of published accounts of private medical companies and establishments; contact with trade organisations for the independent hospital companies (for example cleaning, laundry and portering services). In local contacts with the independent sector there can be no substitute for a sound appreciation of the size and plans of local operators, a knowledge which needs to be as detailed as that of the District's own services. It may also be that some new skills will need to be learned. One example of such skills is in the area of finance and accounting. Few administrators in the NHS are familiar with the traditional accounting statements - Balance Sheets, Profit and Loss Accounts and Funds Flow Statements. Yet in considering handing over vital hospital services to private contractors, it is essential that the NHS is able to assess the financial strengths and weaknesses of companies tendering for the contract. There may be a need, therefore, for the training of administrative and finance staff to be widened to incorporate some of the key skills required in managing commercial enterprises.

It should be briefly mentioned, that similar intelligence needs to be gathered about the stance of the Trade Unions. Whilst in reality any negotiations about privatisation will generally be conducted with local officials, the view of these officials may well be influenced by the stance being taken by Trade Unions centrally. To take a few examples, NUPE has published a glossy 'Education and Information Pack' with the title 'KEEP YOUR SERVICES PUBLIC'. The pack, which has been distributed to all local officials, is a comprehensive action plan intended to enable officials to be well briefed about Government and management tactics and recommends ways in which plans for privatisation can be fought. In District X, the response from NUPE to the possibility of privatisation contained many of the statements which appear in the action kit. Likewise, NALGO has mounted a £1m campaign against privatisation and it too has an 'action kit' for its members. The need to gain intelligence about Trade Unions' views is, however, no more than a step towards the necessity to explain the District's position to staff so that the vital ingredient, trust, can be preserved in relationships with staff. District X was conscious of this need when it agreed to union attendance at the meeting of the health authority where the question of privatisation was being discussed.

Control of Private Sector Developments

As was indicated earlier, the scope for a District to control the development of the private sector locally is minimal. Legislation, for example the Health Services Act 1976 and 1980, and Circular HC(80)10 make provision for DHAs to receive and comment on all applications to the Secretary of State for private hospital developments within the scope of the Acts. However, as this legislation excludes three types of developments - non surgical facilitiies, a unit which does not take the aggregate of private hospital beds beyond 120, and applications for expansion of beds by less than 20 per cent of the total bed complement in a three year period - the influence of the individual DHA is obviously severely limited.

A potentially more powerful control exists in the facility for a District to apply for 'Designation Status' for all or part of the District's territory, under Section 17 of the 1980 Act. If granted, this would require the Secretary of State's authorisation for <u>all</u> private hospital developments within the designated areas, regardless of size. However, it is unlikely that designation could be justified or granted, except in parts of London where there are many private facilities and indeed no such designation has been granted to date.

Registration and Inspection of Nursing Homes

But, in the spirit of collaboration, Districts could have a much more powerful mechanism for control and regulation under the procedures for the Registration of Nursing Homes. Historically, Districts have seen this role as a low priority activity, merely the expression of satisfaction with minimum standards of care. Potentially, however, a District could require the private facility to provide detailed information on staff, accommodation, charges, patients treated and operations performed. In addition, the District could lay down standards of facilities, support services, staffing levels and grades which the unit would have to meet in order to become registered with the District.

Robert Maxwell has said (1983):

> 'Left to itself, the private sector will simply provide what the prosperous consumer will buy and that could quite quickly undermine the concept of a national service ..... To assume that the private sector can do nothing for the public good is only a little less foolish than to assume that it is innately more efficient than the NHS'.

Collaboration on Planning

A positive approach to collaboration would require the establishment of a dialogue with the local private sector. Certainly the circular on Contractual Arrangements [HC(81)1] provides a context within which such a dialogue could take place:

'The Secretary of State hopes that such cooperation and assistance will develop to include consultation at the early planning stages of (independent sector) developments. In the areas where new NHS development is proposed, it is to the advantage of both the NHS and the independent sector to discuss proposals at as early a stage as possible'.

But this exhortation to voluntary collaboration is founded on a general hope rather than a successful history of NHS collaboration with other organisations. Indeed, even in instances where collaboration is a statutory requirement, for example with local authorities, experience has been, at best, mixed. This is not to decry either the effort or the skill of NHS management but rather to emphasise the importance of developing skills in the management of inter-organisational relations. Indeed, it could be argued that a major task for NHS managers in the 1980s may well be regulation of the moving boundaries between the public and private sectors.

Issues for Negotiation

Whilst the above refers to the process of collaboration, what of the substantive issues for discussion? Firstly, it is clear that the NHS retains the responsibility for the wide social policy aspects of health care, for example the objective of equal access to health care for those of equal need. Robert Maxwell's sound advice above suggests the need for the NHS locally to indicate to the private sector the possibilities for cooperation in other than the high technology acute sector, for example in developing services for the mentally ill, the handicapped and the elderly. It could of course be argued that if such areas were profitable, the private sector would already have entered this market. However, this may be rather a restrictive view of future possibilities, because it is possible to contemplate the NHS as the customer - not only in the case of existing services provided by the public sector, but also of services designed specifically to meet the local needs of the NHS. It should also be said that if such innovation became a reality, then it would be a powerful counter to those who see the private sector as 'creaming off' the easier, more lucrative work from the NHS.

A second issue for substantive discussion would be the acute sector itself and the scale and type of local private development which would complement NHS services. There is little evidence yet to show that the private sector has consulted with the NHS on local needs. It has generally attacked the profitable private market for acute clinical services, which has had a number of undesirable effects. For example, the approach has accelerated the shift towards high technology, expensive medicine leading to complaints from the insurance companies, rapid rises in factor costs to the whole health care industry and hampering of the development of non technological aspects of care, both because of lack of finance and because of their diminished importance and prestige. At local level a close partnership might require a joint understanding of the priorities for acute services which in many cases would require the private sector to develop 'bread and butter' services which improve the quality and quantity of basic acute services to the local population. This sort of understanding would be extremely hard to reach but might be the only way of preventing the emergence of a two tier health service - a modern privately owned acute sector for the relatively well off and an NHS which is a safety net for the private sector, the provider of low status services for the long stay patients, under-funded and with low staff and patient morale.

Yet another substantive area of discussion would be the need for an adequate contribution by the private sector towards the training of health care staff. To an extent, the private sector itself has recognised that 'poaching' of staff does not help its image in the public mind. A positive role for the NHS at local level would be to examine ways in which an operational and financial commitment can be obtained from the private sector towards training. Joint training schemes, whereby staff from each sector receive part of their training in the other, would do much to dispel the many myths on both sides whilst at the same time adding to the local pool of trained staff. There is at present a significant difference in the terms and conditions of staff in the two sectors and there is, therefore, a role also for the Central Government department in exploring the possibility of a better alignment.

Contractual Arrangements

Turning now to contractual arrangements for non clinical services, even health authorities sympathetic to the possibility have not been helped by hastily compiled guidance and ill conceived 'model' contracts. There is little doubt that health authorities will need considerable help in the mechanics of privatisation but it is important that central actions do not make the task even more difficult than it is. It would be true to say that the recent draft circular [DA(83)14] has put back the cause of privatisation by many months.

However, there is now little alternative for health authorities but to undertake a close examination of the costs of providing non clinical services. The task is not easy given the accounting systems in the NHS and the very considerable staff time which will be required. These constraints mean that a selective approach will be essential depending on local circumstances. In District X for example, attention is being given first to cleaning services. Also, given the many pitfalls identified earlier, it would be wise for Districts to make haste slowly. It is vital that authorities are seen to be undertaking a fair comparison of costs against private sector tenders. The duty lies on a health authority, in the interests of good financial management and good employee relations, that its own managers of non clinical services are given the financial and administrative support necessary to enable them to submit a tender on which a fair financial comparison might be based.

Assuming that an authority has reached the tendering stage, it would be wise, given the many pitfalls, to consider 'privatising' services initially in a small hospital unit, if one exists within the District. There is very little substitute for experience in this complex and sensitive field and it is vital that the District has an escape route if the contract goes wrong for any reason. Success, however, would not automatically mean a wholesale transition to contractual arrangements, even if this were possible in theory, which is generally not the case. However, experience of managing a small contract for a period of time will doubtless identify numerous lessons for further such arrangements.

Equipment

The Guardian recently reported an arrangement whereby the independent sector had purchased an expensive piece of medical equipment for installation in an NHS hospital. Under the arrangement, the NHS would bear the running costs and the independent sector would have access to the equipment for a proportion of this time. There can be little doubt that similar joint funding and joint use arrangements have wide potential for benefitting both NHS patients and the independent sector.

Concluding Comment

This final Section has identified some of the ways in which the NHS and the independent medical sector might collaborate for the benefit of all - for we all need health care at one time or another. But the list is by no means exhaustive and the task initially is not easy. The fundamental issue is the need for a change in attitude within the NHS towards a positive and deliberate approach to examining the opportunities which collaboration with the independent sector can offer. The suggestions in this Section would then be merely a glimpse of what imaginative collaboration could offer. As has been demonstrated, the intermesh between the public and private sector is already extensive and close - what is now necessary is controlled exploitation of new possibilities.

8 Summary of possible actions for the NHS

It will have been evident that the debate about privatisation in medical care is topical. The final paragraphs of this monograph are being written as the new Conservative Government, returned to Parliament with a landslide majority, is picking up the levers of power which were temporarily on 'neutral' during the election campaign.

The evidence following the election would appear to bear out the thesis that privatisation will be a factor the NHS will have to cope with sooner rather than later. The Guardian of 1 July 1983 carried the front page headline: 'Fowler Slams Breaks on NHS Growth'. The article went on to say that the Government is telling health authorities to plan on the basis of 0.5 per cent real growth per annum for the next ten years - some authorities would receive slightly more and some less on the basis of the equalisation formula. The announcement brought immediate and fierce attacks from the Opposition and other quarters that the announcement proved the existence of the Government's 'hidden agenda' to dismantle the NHS and to hand over its most lucrative elements to the private sector.

In the previous Chapters, it was demonstrated that the NHS can no longer assume that the private sector will remain of peripheral significance. It was further argued that, in order to ensure that the NHS can continue to meet the high objectives for which it was established, those within it need to take a pro-active stance towards collaboration with the private sector. This Chapter summarises some of the possible actions and approaches which might be available to the NHS.

Possible Action at National Level

1 Chairmen of RHAs should now attempt to keep privatisation high on the agenda on their discussions with ministers. The objective should be to ensure that ministers are fully aware of the impact of privatisation on the NHS. This will require good communication channels within the NHS to ensure that chairmen of RHAs are fully briefed on the local and general impact on the NHS of private sector activity.

2 The respective National Associations of health authorities and community health councils also need to take up the debate so that the voice of the 'providers' and 'consumers' can be registered. It may

well be that the voices are not in harmony, but either way, the opportunities for adjustment by the two sectors are likely to be increased.

3 At the national level attention needs to be turned firstly to a fairer contribution to the training of health care personnel and secondly to a better match between the terms and conditions of employment between the two sectors.

Possible Action at the Local Level

1 Local health authorities would now be well advised to undertake a comprehensive audit of the local private sector - its strengths and weaknesses.

2 A serious attempt could be made to test the demand for amenity beds - first by considering whether they are located in the most appropriate hospitals and secondly by publicising their availability.

3 Quality of patient care can be judged by the medical and nursing care, by the quality of support services and finally staff attitudes. There would appear to be scope for change and improvement at least in the latter two elements.

4 Pay beds can constitute an important source of income as well as enabling senior medical staff to remain in close proximity to NHS patients. Authorities should consider how best to ensure the continued use of such facilities - by a management arrangement with the private sector or by improving the standard of fixtures, equipment and fittings.

5 Much closer attention needs to be paid to the task of registering independent sector establishments. The vetting of establishments to ensure they meet service standards would prevent the danger of 'cowboy' operators entering the industry.

6 It may well be that the independent sector could be channelled towards providing services which the NHS is unable to provide up to necessary levels. The prospect of long and medium term contractual arrangements might act as incentive to the independent sector.

7 Reference has already been made to the need for a more equitable arrangement to meet staff training costs.

8 There might well be opportunities for the NHS to seek to share the costs of the expensive medical equipment through a joint use arrangement.

9 In relation to the non clinical services a 'hard nosed' assessment of NHS costs is now urgent. The sooner the technicalities of tendering are grasped the sooner the facts about relative competitive costs can be assessed.

10 Good employee relations practice suggests the need to involve staff and unions in the discussion about privatisation from the earliest possible stage. The cost and staffing comparisons need to be fair but importantly, need to be seen to be fair.

REFERENCES

ABEL-SMITH B (1976): 'Value for Money in Health Services': Heinemann Educational Books Ltd.

ADAM SMITH INSTITUTE (1981): 'Health and the Public Sector: Report to the Minister of Health'.

ASSOCIATION OF HEALTH SERVICE TREASURERS (1981): 'Use of Commercially Provided Services in the NHS'.

BUNKER J P (1974): 'Risks and Benefits of Surgery. In: Taylor D (ed) 'Benefits and Risks in Medical Care', Office of Health Economics.

BUPA, PPP, WPA: Annual Reports and Accounts.

DHSS (1975) Circular DS 267/75: 'Separation of Private Practice from NHS Hospitals: HMSO.

DHSS (1981) Circular HC (80) 10: 'Private Practice in Health Service Hospitals': HMSO.

DHSS (1981) Circular HC (81) 1: 'Contractual Arrangements': HMSO.

DHSS (1980) Circular HC (80) 8: 'Patients First': HMSO.

DHSS (1983) Circular DA (83) 14: 'NHS Support Services - Contracting Out': HMSO.

HEALTH SERVICES BOARD (1977): 'Common Waiting Lists for NHS and Private Patients in NHS Hospitals: Report': HMSO.

HORNE D A (1982): 'Contractual Arrangements: NHS Use of the Private Sector': British Medical Journal: 3 April.

JACQUES E (1976): 'A General Theory of Bureaucracy': Heinemann.

KIRK R (1982): 'Defusing the Private Practice Powder Keg': Health and Social Services Journal, 25 November: pp 1408-9.

KLEIN R (1980): 'Ideology, Class and the National Health Service': King's Fund Project Paper No RC4, March.

LEE DONALDSON ASSOCIATES: 'UK Private Medical Care, Provident Scheme Statistics 1980: London': Lee Donaldson Associates.

MAXWELL R J (1983): 'Money and Management: The NHS in the 1980s': Hospital and Health Services Review, March.

MAXWELL R J (1981): 'Health and Wealth': Lexington Books.

NHS CONSULTANTS ASSOCIATION (1981): 'What's Good About the NHS?: A Discussion Document': London.

NUPE (1983): Letter of 12 April 1983 to the Chairman of District X Health Authority, commenting on privatisation proposals.

OECD (1977): 'Public Expenditure on Health': OECD, Paris.

POWELL J E (1975): 'Medicine and Politics': Pitman Medical Publishing.

REGISTERED NURSING HOMES ASSOCIATION (1982/83): 'Reference Book': Registered Nursing Homes Association.

ROYAL COMMISSION ON THE NHS (1979): Chairman Sir Alec Merrison: HMSO.

THE TIMES HEALTH SUPPLEMENT (1981): 'Private GP Service Closes': Report: 4 December.

VAUGHAN G (1979): Letter from Minister of Health to Chairmen of Health Authorities on 'Cooperation Between the NHS and the Private Sector and the Balance Between Them': 25 June : DHSS.

Appendix 1

CHANGES PLANNED TOWARDS PRIVATISATION

	Asset Sales	Privatisation	Performance Targets	Completion Plan	Spending
BNOC	Yes	No	Yes	No	Yes
Electricity	No	No	Yes	Yes	Yes
Gas	Yes	No	Yes	Yes	Yes
Coal	No	No	Yes	No	Yes
Freight	Yes	No	No	No	No
National Bus	No	No	Yes	Yes	No
British Rail	Yes	Yes	Yes	No	No
Docks	Yes	No	Yes	No	No
British Airports	No	No	Yes	No	No
British Airways	Yes	No	Yes	No	No
Telecom	No	Yes	Yes	Yes	Yes
Post Office	No	No	Yes	Yes	No
British Aerospace	Yes	No	No	No	No
British Shipbuilders	No	No	No	No	No
British Steel	Yes	Yes	Yes	No	Yes
BL	Yes	No	No	No	No
British Technology	Yes	No	No	No	No

Source: Daily Telegraph 18 January 1982.

Appendix 2

AMENITY AND PRIVATE BEDS BY NHS REGION (31 DECEMBER 1979)

RHA	Av Daily No of beds (including Amenity and Private)	Amenity Beds	Private Beds
Northern	25,305	216	56
Yorkshire	29,946	262	140
Trent	31,741	283	130
East Anglia	13,094	49	90
N W Thames	27,904	88	339
N E Thames	29,443	163	278
S E Thames	28,408	140	263
S W Thames	26,242	328	156
Wessex	19,021	177	99
Oxford	13,664	103	164
S Western	24,456	136	78
West Midlands	36,263	291	181
Mersey	21,982	200	67
North Western	30,812	194	170
Total England	358,252	2,630	2,211

Appendix 3

HOSPITAL AND COMMUNITY SERVICES: CONTRACTING OUT
ENGLAND 1980/81

	Total Revenue Expenditure £m	External Contracts £m	% of Total
Total, all Services	6,551	163	2.5
Patient Care	4,037	45	1.1
Homes and Hospitals	-	27	-
Maintenance of Technical Equipment	-	18	-
General Services	2,216	118	5.3
Catering	316	1	0.3
Portering	126	0	0.0
Domestic/Cleaning	375	10	2.6
Linen/Laundry	146*	7	4.8
Transport	30*	7	23.0
Estate Management	637	93	15.0
of which			
- Engineering maintenance		43	
- Building maintenance		47	
- Gardening and farming		3	
Other	586	-	-
Other, including ambulance	298	0	0.0

* Hospitals only

Sources: NHS Appropriation Accounts:
Second Report of the Social Services Committee; Session 1981/82 Vol II.

Appendix 4

BUPA, PPP, WPA - KEY STATISTICS

Year	Persons Insured (000s)	Subscribers (000s)	Subscriptions Earned (£m)	Benefits Incurred (£m)
1955	585	274	1.83	1.54
1956	680	318	2.26	1.92
1957	755	354	2.76	2.32
1958	825	387	3.28	2.76
1959	895	419	3.85	3.24
1960	995	467	4.47	3.76
1961	1,070	504	5.19	4.36
1962	1,165	546	6.00	5.22
1963	1,250	587	6.97	6.23
1964	1,345	632	7.99	7.13
1965	1,445	680	9.12	8.02
1966	1,565	735	10.68	9.35
1967	1,670	784	12.52	10.86
1968	1,770	831	14.45	12.22
1969	1,887	886	17.34	14.86
1970	1,982	930	20.35	16.89
1971	2,102	986	23.79	19.74
1972	2,196	1,021	28.90	24.49
1973	2,265	1,064	36.24	29.24
1974	2,334	1,096	45.20	36.24
1975	2,315	1,087	54.92	45.59
1976	2,251	1,057	70.57	53.15
1977	2,254	1,057	90.72	64.68
1978	2,388	1,118	105.06	67.68
1979	2,765	1,292	122.06	83.96
1980	3,577	1,647	154.34	127.61

KEY POINTS FROM 1981 REPORT AND ACCOUNTS

	BRITISH UNITED PROVIDENT ASSOCIATION	PRIVATE PATIENTS PLAN	WESTERN PROVIDENT ASSOCIATION	BRISTOL CONTRIBUTORY WELFARE ASSOCIATION	CRUSADER INSURANCE PLC (GROUP HEALTH ACCOUNT)
Established	1947	1940	1939	1935	n.a.
Head Office	Provident House, Essex St London WC2	Eynsham House, Crescent Rd. Tunbridge Wells	Culverhouse, Culver St Bristol	Bristol Hse Victoria Street Bristol	Reigate, Surrey
Branch Offices/Sales Centres	22	9	5	0	36
Employees	1,892	447	80 (est)	35 (est)	approx. 50
Number of Registrations	1,396,000	353,000	114,000(Private Treatment Scheme) c 100,000(Health Service Scheme)	c 20,000(Private Patients Scheme) c 15,000(Hospital Contributory Scheme)	c 40,000
Subscription Income(1)	£143,455,000	£49,841,184	£9,663,503	£2,396,066	£4,000,000(approx)
Benefits Paid(1)	£142,344,000	£44,975,147	£8,307,136	£1,894,299	not known
Claims rate after(before) transfers from reserve	86.3% (99.2%)	86.3%(90.2%)	86.0%	79.1%	95% (approx)
Subscriber benefit reserve	£39,447,000	£3,100,000	)no corresponding provision	)no corresponding provision	n.a.
Amount of transfer	£18,472,000	£2,300,009	)	)	
General reserves(3) (% of sub income)	£72,704,000(50.7%)	£24,893,712(49.9%)	£3,459,507 (35.8%)	£,730,893(72.2%)	n.a.
Proportion of subscription income spent on admin and development	15.0%	12.7%	12.6%	12.2%	n.a.
Schemes currently available	Group Bulk Protection Scheme Optional BPS Company Care Large BUPACARE International Individual BUPACARE Unit Scheme Undergrad & Students Schools International Worldwide Travel Scheme BMA Scheme Cash Scheme BUCS(2)	Group Company Masterplan Company Masterplan) International) Individual Family Masterplan Family Masterplan International Private Hospital Plan Young Persons Plan BMA Scheme Dental Plan	Group Supercover Individual Supercover Contributory Scheme Health Service Scheme	Group Private Patients Plan Individual Private Patients Scheme Contributory Scheme Maxi Plan Double Maxi Plan Senior Citizen Plan	Group Medical Aid Plan1 Medical Aid Plan2 Medical Aid Plan3 Individual None (most classes of insurance transacted)
Charitable Donations	£727,000 to NNHT £231,000 to other Charities plus:£6.5m loan to NNHT £2.25m loan to other charities	£82,857 to NNHT £61,072 to Eynsham Trust £3,142 to other charities plus:£1.5m loan to Eynsham Trust. £3.0m to other charitable organisations	£52,822 to WPA Medical Charities Fund £500 to other organisations plus:£84,214 loan to WPA Medical Charities Fund	£5,000 to BCWA Charitable Trust	£23,651

(1) Before transfers from reserve (2) Not included in subscription and benefit figures (3) 'General Reserves' are total reserves minus subscriber benefit reserve, reserves for unearned premiums and outstanding claims, etc. (4) Most of this information gained from a meeting with Crusader in March 1982.

Appendix 6

1982 NALGO ANNUAL CONFERENCE

TEXT OF RESOLUTION ON PRIVATE MEDICINE

'Conference is increasingly concerned at the growing number of applications for private hospitals and pay beds which has been encouraged by the policies of the Government and has resulted in a drain upon the resources of the National Health Service.

Conference deprecates the Government's failure to heed the call of the trade union movement to maintain and improve the previously high standards of the National Health Service and deplores its apparent intent to institute a system of health care which discriminates against the less privileged members of our society.

Conference reaffirms its total opposition to a health service based upon the principle of ability to pay, and in view of the ineffectiveness of recent measures to defend the National Health Service, urges Branches to refuse to cooperate with applications for private hospitals and allocation of pay beds, and instructs the National Executive Council to:

(1) give its full support to Branches taking this action;

(ii) take immediate steps to publicise, both to NALGO members and the general public, the inadequacies of private health care and combat the misconception that private insurance can provide complete and indefinite medical cover;

(iii) take the initiative in the TUC to ensure that a more positive and radical programme of action is adopted to obtain the restoration of the National Health Service to a position where it can meet the needs of society and absorb all health care into the public sector'.

Appendix 7

ADVERTISEMENT FOR INDEPENDENT HOSPITAL UNIT

!!!! PRIVATE SURGERY AND MEDICAL CARE !!!!

Why wait months for hospital treatment when we can help to relieve your worry and pain.

LOW FEES, EARLY ADMISSION

Our qualified consultant surgeon (FRCS) whom we employ full-time will be available to see you and undertake your care personally at your own private hospital registered with District X Health Authority.

EARLY ADMISSIONS AND CONSULTATIONS
EXAMPLES OF TREATMENT OFFERED

General Surgery		Fees
Varicose Veins	from	£260
Hernia Repair	from	£340
Piles	from	£480
Prostate	from	£480

Cosmetic-Surgery		Fees
Breast Enlargement	from	£739
Nose Reshaping	from	£676
Facelift	from	£978
Eyebag Removal	from	£489

AND MOST OTHER OPERATIONS

WE LOOK FORWARD TO CARING FOR YOU

THE SISTER MARY PRIVATE CLINIC

Telephone: Address:

Appendix 8

DEPARTMENT OF HEALTH AND SOCIAL SECURITY

Alexander Fleming House
Elephant & Castle
London SE1 6BY
Telephone 01-407-5522

From the Minister for Health

20 August 1981

Dear Chairman

EFFICIENCY AND CONTRACT SERVICES

Earlier this year the Department issued a formal circular [HC(81)1] about contractual arrangements with private hospitals. This letter concerns the use of commercial contractors for other NHS purposes.

As you know, I believe that the use of a good contractor, under a carefully drawn and properly controlled contract, can be an excellent way of increasing efficiency, thus freeing money for patient care. I have therefore been disappointed to hear that some Authorities have not responded constructively to approaches from commercial companies, notably from the cleaning industry. Others, I am glad to say, have been more positive.

It would be helpful if you could let me know what possibilities your own Authority has considered, and what progress you have made. I am particularly interested in domestic and laundry services, maintenance of buildings and vehicles, security services and transport services. These seem likely to offer the greatest scope for contractual arrangements. But I am interested also in catering, computers, any pharmaceutical or other manufacturing for which there is an alternative commercial supply, and indeed any other services where you may see scope.

I have myself had useful meetings with representatives of the cleaning and laundry industries. Both were rightly concerned that the alternatives should be considered on the basis of a full and realistic comparison of costs. The cleaning industry impressed on me their readiness to meet the specialised needs of NHS units of all sizes. The laundry industry are particularly interested in opportunities for new investment, and I would urge any Authority which is contemplating large scale expenditure on a laundry to consider the commercial alternatives before deciding. Likewise, any proposal to invest resources in manufacturing facilities (eg for the production of sterile solutions) should proceed only if the Authority is convinced that the products cannot be obtained from other sources.

Use of contractors might be particularly appropriate to provide services in newly commissioned buildings. I should be grateful if you could say in your reply to what extent contractors will be used in any new development which your Authority will be responsible for running.

I am writing in identical terms to all RHAs, AHAs and BG Chairmen.

Yours sincerely

DR GERARD VAUGHAN

Appendix 9

EXTRACT FROM PAPER ON CONTRACTING OUT CLEANING SERVICES IN DISTRICT X

SUMMARY OF THE CASE FOR AND AGAINST THE EMPLOYMENT OF 'HOTEL SERVICES' CONTRACTORS IN THE NHS.

Points for

1 The larger companies have the specialism, expertise and experience to undertake any kind of domestic work and are capable of achieving high standards even with large scale operations. An Association of Health Service Treasurers report earlier this year indicates many examples of very good services being provided.

2 Lower costs than direct labour may be achieved by spreading managerial and supervisory overheads over a large volume of labour. Economies of scale also apply with the larger contractors with regard to the purchase of materials and equipment.

3 Contract cleaning is promoted as being particularly relevant where problems of staff recruitment/retention and of effective management/supervision are being experienced. Experience suggests that costs are of only equal significance to the other problem areas.

4 The costs of contract services are known and fixed in advance which facilitates budgeting and the potentially damaging effects of high sickness and absence levels.

5 Intense competition from other contractors encourages maintenance of high standards. A contract can be terminated easily if the standards fall below those stipulated in the agreement.

6 Contractors encourage cross pollination of ideas with new methods of working to improve efficiency.

7 Although opposition from trades unions is normally to be expected, experience has demonstrated that problems are normally resolved very quickly and harmonious relations with contractors are in fact the rule.

8 The use of contractors largely frees the NHS from the administrative problems of providing support services and enables more time to be devoted to the task of its primary function of health care.

Points Against

1 Managers of support services have greater overall expertise to solve problems than contractors and are able to call on the same range of specialist advisors as are available to the contractors.

2 On the crucial question of staff interests, employment by contractor cannot reproduce all the benefits associated with public sector employment, especially job security and inflation linked pensions.

3 Several hospitals, having had experience of contractors, have reverted to a directly managed service on the grounds of inadequate standards or cost.

4 Especially in smaller health authorities, there may be no one with the necessary detailed knowledge and experience of cleaning techniques, standards, procedures, equipment and materials to ensure that the service being bought is actually being provided and that it is sufficiently sensitive to meet the changing needs of hospital users.

5 Where a contractor is given notice to terminate, there is inevitably a falling off of standards as staff leave and management loses interest, which is unacceptable in a hospital situation.

6 Where NHS management takes a positive position on standards and demands them from its own organisation to ensure the effective use of resources, a cost effective service can be provided which is likely to be cheaper than a contractor.

7 The employment of contractors could mean the loss of integrated ward teams, reduced standards as a result of cost cutting where a contract has been mispriced, and a waste of the investment in management and supervisory training.

8 The amount of detailed preparatory work, especially for a large hospital contract, is immense if the tenders are to be invited on a valid basis and if the existing direct labour service is to be accurately costed out for comparison purposes.

9 Only 40 NHS units are currently on contract domestic services. Can the other 1,960 all be wrong?